ORTHOPAEDIC
TRACTION
MANUAL

ORTHOPAEDIC TRACTION MANUAL

Andrew F. Brooker, Jr., M.D.
Chief, Department of Orthopaedics
Baltimore City Hospitals
Associate Professor of Orthopaedic Surgery
Johns Hopkins University
School of Medicine

Gerhard Schmeisser, M.D.
Professor and Associate Director
Department of Orthopaedic Surgery
Johns Hopkins University
School of Medicine

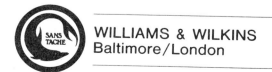

WILLIAMS & WILKINS
Baltimore/London

Copyright ©, 1980
The Williams & Wilkins Company
428 E. Preston Street
Baltimore, MD 21202, U.S.A.

Made in the United States of America

Library of Congress Cataloging in Publication Data

Brooker, Andrew F
  The orthopaedic traction manual.

  Includes index.
  1. Orthopedic traction—Handbooks, manuals, etc.
I. Schmeisser, Gerhard, joint author. II. Title.
[DNLM: 1. Traction—Handbooks. WE190 B872o]
RD736.T7B76   617'.3   79-25268
ISBN 0-683-01074-3

Composed and printed at the
Waverly Press, Inc.
Mt. Royal and Guilford Aves.
Baltimore, MD 21202, U.S.A.

Dedication

To Doctor Robert A. Robinson, Professor of Orthopaedic Surgery, The Johns Hopkins Hospital, 1953 to 1979.

A.B. & G.S.

Preface

At a time when surgical treatment of most fractures is being enthusiastically practiced and when new casting or bracing materials are available, it seems superficially inappropriate to write a manual of orthopaedic traction techniques. In fact, the ability to intelligently and correctly apply traction is one of the most basic skills. Every practicing orthopaedic surgeon will see patients whose injuries are too severe or fractures too comminuted for prudent surgical correction. He will also encounter the injured child who heals quickly without surgery or the infected joint replacement that requires a period of rest in traction. Perhaps most important of all, the orthopaedic resident must be exposed to the techniques of traction since it gives him an alternative method of treating nearly every major fracture. Anyone of us may employ traction when we choose to avoid surgery or perhaps find ourselves practicing in circumstances devoid of modern operating rooms.

Orthopaedic traction, if properly utilized, is a safe and rewarding alternative form of treatment. Its potential, however, is frequently not fully appreciated because success with traction depends on a high level of understanding of its principles and cooperation in its practice by all members of the patient care team.

Thus, the purpose of this book is to facilitate the better use of traction by presenting the pertinent principles, equipment, method of application, and assembly in such a fashion as to be meaningful to all members of the hospital staff involved in patient care. We have omitted certain techniques such as traction of the hand or forefoot since they are seldom employed and are frequently very individualized. We have also omitted traction techniques to correct joint contractures and congenital dislocation of the hip since methods used for the treatment of these clinical problems can be adapted easily from principles presented within this text.

The authors will be especially pleased if this manual finds its way into the nurses' stations, emergency rooms, and the hands of the students of orthopaedic surgery and its related disciplines. The book's size, binding, and format were selected to meet the practical needs of this group. Line drawing illustrations are used in the interest of both clarity and economy.

Acknowledgments

The authors would like to acknowledge the enthusiasm and dedication of Mrs. Halina Kowalczyk in the preparation of this text. In addition the cooperation of William and Wilkins as well as the artistic effort of Mrs. Diane Abeloff made this book possible.

A.B. & G.S.

Contributor

Vernon T. Tolo, M.D.
Chief, Pediatric Orthopaedic Surgery
Johns Hopkins University
School of Medicine
Director of Scoliosis Clinics
Johns Hopkins University
School of Medicine

Contents

Preface..vii

Acknowledgments...viii

Contributor...x

Objectives and Limitations..3

Chapter 1: ORTHOPAEDIC EQUIPMENT..................................5
           Beds and Frames..5

Chapter 2: KNOTS...11

Chapter 3: SPINAL TRACTION.......................................15

           Cervical Traction.....................................15
              Head Halter Traction for Relief of Neck Pain
              or Temporary Splinting.............................15
              Gardner Tongs - Skeletal Traction for Cervical
              Spine Trauma.......................................18
              Crutchfield Tong Traction..........................21
              Outpatient Cervical Traction for Management of
              Chronic Neck Pain..................................22
              Halo Ring Traction.................................23

           Traction for Spinal Deformities.......................29
              Cotrel Dynamic Traction............................30
              Halo Femoral Traction..............................30
              Halo Pelvic Traction...............................32
              Halo Suspension Device.............................36

           Lumbar Traction.......................................38
              Inpatient Pelvic Belt for Acute Back Pain..........38
              Home Pelvic Traction...............................38

Chapter 4: UPPER EXTREMITY TRACTION..............................43

           Skin Traction and its Limitations.....................43
           Simple Forearm Skin Traction..........................43
           Double Skin Traction: Forearm and Upper Arm...........46
           Dunlop's Technique for Supracondylar Fractures........48
           Overhead Olecranon Pin Traction.......................50
           Lateral Olecranon Pin Traction........................53
           Metacarpal Pin Traction - Reduction Technique.........54
           Finger Trap Traction..................................56

1

Chapter 5: TRACTION FOR PELVIC OR ACETABULAR FRACTURES............ 61

                Pelvic Sling Suspension...................... 61
                Upper Femoral Skeletal Traction.............. 62

Chapter 6: LOWER EXTREMITY TRACTION............................... 67

                Traction for Femoral Fractures................ 67
                Split Russell's Traction (Backs with a Sling). 69
                Knee and Hip Exerciser........................ 71
                Low Angle Bryants or Bilateral Uphill Backs... 72
                Ninety-90 Degree Traction of the Distal Femur. 73
                Distal Femoral Traction in Extension.......... 77
                Proximal Tibial Traction in Extension........ 79
                Balanced Suspension with Splint and Pearson
                Attachment.................................... 81
                Balanced Suspension with Double Slings........ 89
                Neufeld Traction (Balanced Suspension in a Long
                Leg Cast)..................................... 93
                Distal Tibial Skeletal Traction.............. 94
                Calcaneal Traction........................... 98
                Transmetatarsal Suspension................... 98

Objectives and Limitations

Although traction is used to rest and protect an injured joint, to enforce bed rest for low back pain, and to immobilize the hip following removal of an infected total joint replacement, its usual purpose is to align fractures and to maintain this position until healing occurs. With any fracture, the same goals may be obtained by various combinations of the techniques: manual closed reduction, plaster cast immobilization, open surgical reduction, internal or external metallic fixation, and traction. Experienced judgment is required in making the best selection of these alternatives and, on occasion, appreciating the advantages of combining several approaches.

Treatment of any fracture with traction techniques has certain advantages. In avoiding surgery, the injured bone is exposed to less risk of infection and is not devascularized in a surgical dissection which may retard healing . Additionally, traction allows more joint mobility and muscle exercises than is permitted in plaster encasement.

The major disadvantage of traction is prolonged recumbency and the increased risk of thromboembolic disease. These risks preclude the use of traction techniques in certain patients. However, with modern prophylactic approaches to thromboembolic risks, early physical therapy to avoid contractures, and vigorous nursing care, traction continues to offer a sound alternative to most of the difficult problems existing in orthopaedics.

CHAPTER 1

Orthopaedic Equipment

Beds and Frames

Beds for traction should have the same positional adjustment capabilities as most modern hospital beds. They should also have structural characteristics which permit rigid and secure attachment of traction framing.

Positional adjustments especially appropriate for traction patients include not only the usual back, knee, and leg adjustments, but also tilt adjustments, head down (Trendelenberg), and foot down (reverse Trendelenberg). Back, knee, and leg adjustments are necessary to establish and maintain specific patient and limb position whereby fracture fragment alignment can be obtained and held while union occurs. Tilt adjustments are necessary to obtain countertraction and frequently avoid need for shock blocks. High-low bed movements are seldom useful for patients in traction apparatus, except when Bradford frames are used as described in the next paragraph. Usually, these beds should be fully elevated to facilitate bedside care. When certain traction systems are used, a variety of traction system malalignments may occur if either the level of the bed or one of the positional adjustments is altered; therefore, the bed should be provided with master switches located at the foot of the bed, out of the patient's reach. These master switches enable medical personnel to deactivate the patient's bed controls. Otherwise, it may be desirable to disconnect the bed's main power plug from the wall socket after appropriate posture is achieved.

The ideal bed for traction treatment of patients with severe or multiple musculoskeletal injuries is an electrically powered hospital bed with a rectangular Bradford frame and with high-low mattress and spring adjustability (Fig. 1). It should be designed with a platform frame of fixed height and to which the lower ends of the vertical poles of a 4-pole traction assembly are permanently attached. The bed design must allow the mattress and springs to move up and down on top of the platform frame and independently of the traction assembly. When used with a Bradford frame attached at each corner to one of the vertical poles, the mattress and springs can be lowered while the patient's weight is supported by the Bradford frame. This feature enables bedpan placement or bed linen change with minimal disturbance of the patient or his traction system. A Bradford frame is not compatible with back, knee, and leg bed adjustments. Usually when the patient is well enough

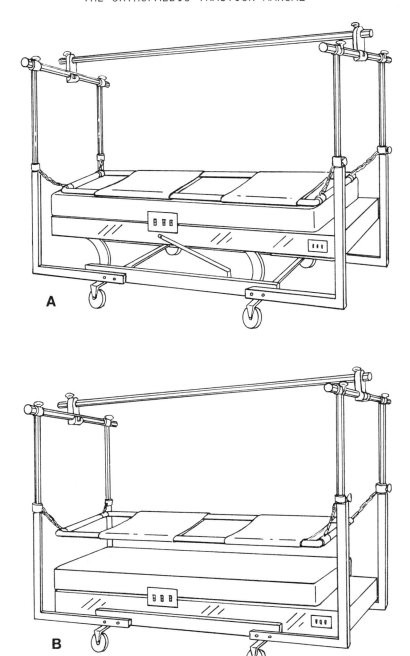

Fig. 1:   The ideal bed for traction treatment of patients with severe
           or multiple musculoskeletal injuries has high-low mattress
           adjustability, a removable Bradford frame, and a permanent
           4-post, fixed height traction frame.

to use these adjustments, the Bradford frame is no longer needed and can be removed.

Although wood beams 2 x 4 inch, ordinary metal pipe, or square tubing can be used successfully for traction frames, octagonal aluminum tubing has been the material most widely used for many years. Poles of this material require little or no maintenance, are light, and can be stored easily, disassembled on a special cart or in a closet large enough to accommodate 8-foot lengths. This material needs little or no maintenance care. A variety of traction pole fittings are available which permit temporary attachment of octagonal pole assemblies to most types of hospital beds. The system with upper and lower toggle clamps as illustrated in Figure 2A, is designed to grasp the headboard and footboard of the bed. When this system is used, the attachments of the headboard and footboard to the bed frame should be examined carefully. Frequently, they consist of several small machine screws which might not sustain the force levels imposed by some traction systems. Proper adjustment of the toggles is important in order to grasp the headboard and footboard tightly enough to avoid slipping. Secure closure of the upper toggle may require considerable muscular effort.

Systems designed to fit the intravenous pole sockets located at each corner of the bed, as illustrated in Figure 2B, are easier to apply and may be more stable. Personnel who are assembling the system should be certain that the sockets are sturdy and securely attached to the bed frame.

Offset, upright poles are available which have been designed to avoid contact of the traction poles with and damage to wall-mounted lights and other fixtures at the head end of the bed. When assembling a traction system with an offset pole, special attention is required to avoid placing traction weights directly over the patient's head. Routing traction lines to the foot end of the bed may be required in order to suspend the weights in locations where they cannot descend onto the patient.

Some beds are designed for the bed frame to shorten or telescope toward the head end as the backrest is elevated (Fig. 2C). This telescoping feature causes the patient's head to remain the same distance from the headboard regardless of the degree of elevation of the backrest. This design has the desirable feature of minimizing displacement of any tubes or electrical wires running from the patient to equipment located near the head of the bed. Longitudinal overhead traction poles which telescope have been designed for these beds. Such a frame should be used with a special diagonal brace at the foot end. In spite of these special frames, bed adjustments of this type are likely to cause maladjustment of some of the more complex traction systems. For this reason, with such systems it is sometimes appropriate either to disengage the telescoping mechanism or to use a different type of bed.

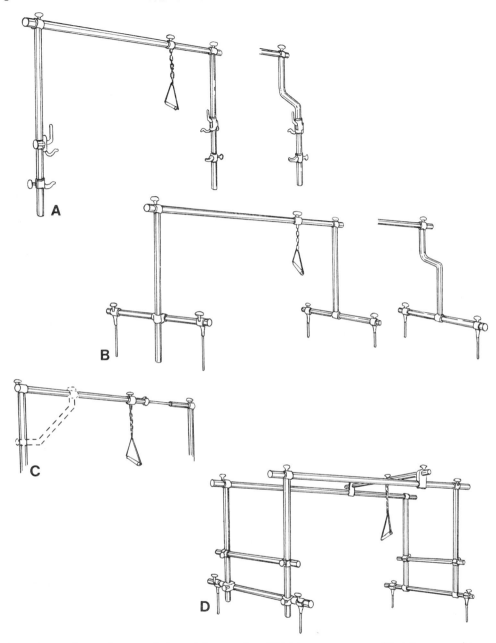

Fig. 2:   A variety of traction pole fittings are available permit-
           ting temporary attachment of octagonal pole assemblies to
           most types of hospital beds. Offset poles at the head end
           are designed to avoid damaging wall-mounted lights.

Fig. 2A: The system with upper and lower clamps grasps the headboard
          and footboard of the bed.
     2B: A system designed to fit intravenous pole sockets at each
          corner of the bed may be more stable.
     2C: Some frames are designed to be compatible with beds designed
          to telescope. They require a special brace at the foot end.
     2D: The most stable assemblies have 4 vertical poles, multiple
          transverse poles, and one or two longitudinal poles.

                    * * * * * * * * *

     The most stable traction frame assemblies have four vertical trac-
tion poles, one at each corner and two horizontal transverse poles which
partially stabilize the vertical poles (Fig. 2D).   Either one or two
longitudinal over-the-bed poles are used to connect the poles at the
head end to those at the foot end, further stabilizing the entire assembly (Fig. 1).   If the system rests on intravenous pole sockets, one
should be certain that they are sturdy and securely attached to the bed
frame.

     Components. Certain features of clamps designed to connect trac-
tion poles together and to various pole accessories deserve special attention. The components of these clamps are frequently aluminum castings with steel hinge pins and steel screw-down fasteners. Failure of
these castings is very rare, but hinge pins occasionally work loose and
screw-down fasteners may abrade the softer contact surgace of the casting, thereby enabling unintentional clamp release. Visual inspection to
detect these problems should be performed whenever assembling or adjusting the equipment.

     Screw-down fasteners may be designed with wing nuts, T-wrenches, or
contoured knobs. Clamps equipped with these knobs are the most comfortable to adjust and are generally the most satisfactory. Clamps on the
ends of vertical support poles should swivel 360 degrees, whereas those
on the ends of short poles used for crossbars should not swivel at all.
Pole clamps with 16 facets are preferrable to those with 8 and enable
attachment in a greater range of positions.

     Pulleys should move freely. Ballbearing ones are usually prefer-
able. Pulley size should be compatible with traction cord thickness,
and dimensional tolerances should not permit the cord to slip between
the sheave and its housing, thereby jamming the pulley. One-eighth inch
or three-sixteenths inch braided nylon cord makes excellent traction
cord. It is strong and cheap and a large quantity is easily stored in
a small space.

     Three different devices are marketed for use as traction weights.
These are water bags, sand bags, and cast iron weights. Sand bags and
cast iron weights are supplied in sizes from 1 to 5 lbs. Water bags can

be filled to appropriate levels for the weight desired and emptied when not in use. When filled, they occupy more space than sand bags or cast iron weights. This is a disadvantage when large traction loads are used. Water bags are usually preferred for home use and sand bags and cast iron weights for institutional use.

CHAPTER 2

Knots

Ideal knots for many traction circumstances are ones which can be tied with one hand while the other hand is occupied holding tension on the traction line or holding a traction weight. Ideal traction knots should be easy to tie, secure, and easy to untie. They should involve minimum lenths of cord. The overhand loop (Fig. 3). and the slip knot (Fig. 4) satisfy these requirements. When a nonsliding loop is desired, the overhand loop may be used. When a sliding loop is desired, the slip knot may be used.

The clove hitch, which can also be tied under tension is frequently useful (Fig. 41). The bowline is a useful nonsliding loop knot; however, it is more difficult to tie under tension.

Since surgeons are generally skillful in tying grannies and squares with one hand, they tend to apply this skill to traction cord. Unfortunately, the result is a knot which runs for an excessive distance along the traction line. It jams pulleys and is tedious to unite.

To prevent unraveling, free ends should always be finished off with an overhand knot or singed with a flame rather than wrapped with adhesive tape. The latter technique is time consuming initially and ultimately untidy. There is no advantage in the similarly messy practice of concealing the knot itself under a wad of tape.

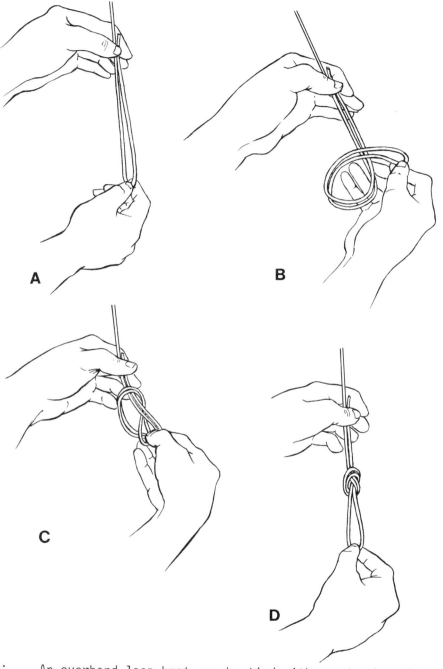

Fig. 3:   An overhand loop knot can be tied with one hand while the
            other holds tension on the line. The loop will not slip.

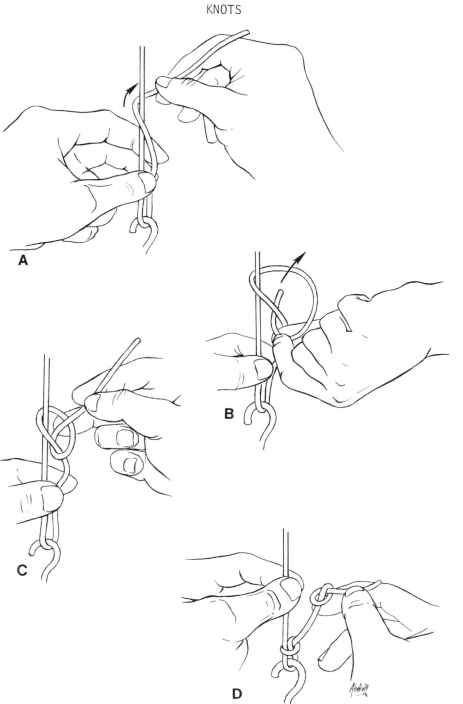

Fig. 4:   A slip knot can be tied with one hand while the other holds
           tension on the line. The loop will tighten.

CHAPTER 3

Spinal Traction

CERVICAL

This term generally applies to various devices that grasp the head and exert traction forces on the cervical spine. They are most commonly used for treating injuries from the atlanto-occipital joint to T-1.

Head Halter Traction

Indications. This type of simple cervical traction is most commonly used for the conservative management of neck pain both in the hospital and as a form of outpatient therapy.

The second most frequent indication for head halter traction is the acutely injured patient where it provides temporary splintage while the neck injury is more fully evaluated and the patient stabilized. Some authors have advised against its use in these patients because of the manipulation necessary to apply the device. We continue to recommend it for these patients but agree that extreme care must be employed.

Application. The head halter may vary in design but generally consists of two pads, one which secures a purchase on the occiput while the other grasps the chin. Each attached loop of cord is designed to lead over the ear and is secured through a metal spreader to the traction line. (Fig. 5)

In the emergency room there is generally a stretcher provided with an attached pulley system. The responsible physician and at least one other person may gently lift the head just enough to slip the head halter into position. Weight is then applied so that the traction line is perfectly parallel to the surface of the stretcher and in line with the cervical spine (Fig. 5A). Weight must never exceed 5 lbs. initially and no flexion or extension force should be caused by the traction until evaluation of the injury is complete. The alert patient will tolerate this form of splintage temporarily, but with increased weight or prolonged traction, the patient will develop discomfort over the jaw. If the head halter is to be continued, adjustment of the weight or realignment of the traction force is required.

In a patient with neck pain, cervicogenic arm, or shoulder pain, application of the head halter can often be accomplished by the patient himself. The traction system is generally attached to the head of the bed so that the patient may have his head slightly elevated (Fig. 6).

15

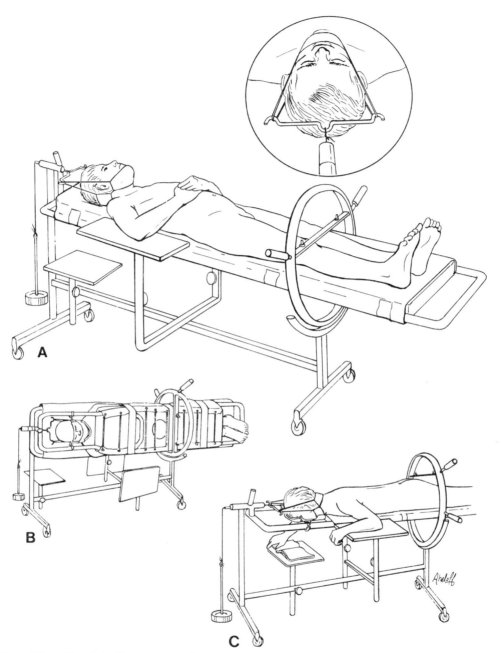

Fig. 5A: Head halter traction on a Stryker frame.
    B: Patient with head halter traction in turning position.
    C: Patient prone.

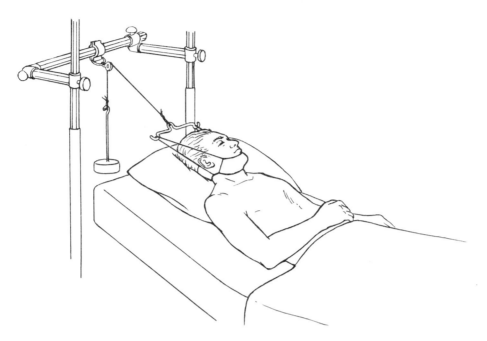

Fig. 6: Frame for head halter traction in hospital bed.

This position is better tolerated by the alert, cooperative patient than
the perfectly flat alignment used in the acutely injured. Because the
halter is designed to get its major purchase on the occipat, the traction line is generally arranged so that a slight flexion force reduces
the pull on the chin. Weights in this circumstance are generally begun
at 5 lbs. and adjusted afterwards according to the patient's response
to the traction weight. In excess of 5 to 7 lbs is seldom tolerated for
prolonged periods.

   Risks. In the acutely injured, excessive manipulation when applying
the head halter traction is a major concern and could obviously aggra-
vate a significant injury causing the patient permanent neurologic damage.

   Unstable injuries of the upper cervical spine are particularly sus-
ceptible to distraction leading to neurologic compromise. For this reason, initial application of weight should never exceed 5 lbs in the
adult. Excessive weight will inevitably cause discomfort at the TM
joint and skin problems in the area over the chin.

   Length of time in traction is also a factor so that the author seldom uses head halter traction continuously for more than 6 to 8 hrs.
Skin problems can develop rapidly. In addition, such head halter de-

vices are cumbersome for nursing care or feeding and poorly tolerated
by alert patients. Head halter traction is clearly contraindicated in
a comatose patient.

Skeletal Traction

Indications. Cervical skeletal traction is used exclusively to
treat the unstable spine. Pull is exerted along the axis of the spine
and these traction forces preserve alignment and volume of the bony canal
protecting the spinal cord. For this reason, its use is limited almost
completely to trauma, fractures or dislocations, and only rarely to tu-
mors where bony stability has been jeopardized.

On rare occasions, skeletal traction is employed to accomplish reduction of cervical facet dislocations, but this is a procedure that requires considerable expertise, and its application exists far beyond the
scope of this book.

There are several currently popular types of tongs used for grasping
the skull and applying cervical skeletal traction. Their indications
are identical. Only the technique of application and the risks involved
vary significantly. The authors have chosen to illustrate the Gardner-
Wells and Crutchfield tongs.

Application Technique for Gardner Tongs. The Gardner tongs are far
easier to apply than either Veneke or Crutchfield tongs and are less
likely to loosen under a prolonged traction load than the Crutchfields.

The patient will generally be supine, protected with either sandbags
or head halter traction. Initially, he is placed on the bed or turning
frame where he will remain for his initial period of hospitalization.
Then, holding the tongs without the sterile inserts initially, the surgeon decides on the area of placement and makes sure that the tongs fit
adequately and clear the head. The tongs should be placed directly
cephalad or above the external auditory meatus approximately in line
with the mastoid process and should just clear the top of the ears
(Fig. 7). This will place them in a longitudinal axis of the spine neu-
tralizing the tendency for flexion or extension forces. They will also
be low caudad enough so that slippage off the top of the skull is unlikely. If anesthesia is indicated, then approximately lcc of 1% xylocaine
is normally instilled after the local area has been shaved and prepped
(Fig. 8). The tongs are held in alignment by an assistant with the
sterile points just touching the skin. When the position is satisfactory, the two screws on either side of the device are turned down simultaneously.

It is essential that the head is supported during this procedure and
that the small indicator on the side of the Gardner device is watched
carefully. As it begins to protrude, approximately 30 lbs of pressure

exists between the two sides of the device. No additional force is required. It is not necessary to make a formal skin incision with this
unit. Having thoroughly engaged the outer table of the skull, traction
is applied by attaching the traction line through the eye at the top of
the tongs. This line is threaded through the turning frame and traction
is applied. The final step in application is obtaining an x-ray of the
skull and cervical spine to ascertain alignment and position of the
tongs. Weights can be adjusted on the basis of x-ray and level of the
defect. In subsequent days, the tongs must be carefully and routinely
cleaned to avoid local infections. Our most successful routine has been
frequent use of peroxide soaked cotton-tipped application to gently de-
bride the pin site with occasional application of alcohol to keep the
metal free of any debris.

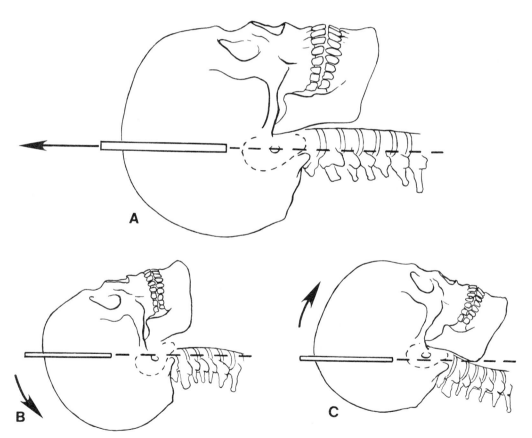

Fig. 7A: Proper alignment for Gardner tongs.
     B: Excessive anterior placement.
     C: Excessive posterior placement.

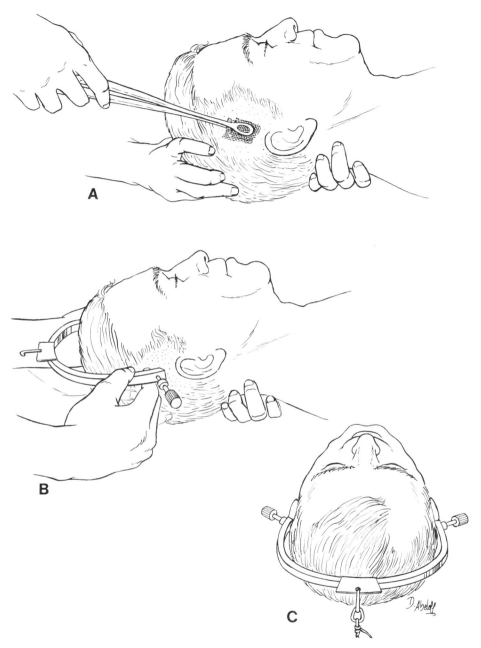

Fig. 8A: Preparation of area for tong application. (Note assistant
          stabilizing head and neck.)
     B: Proper positioning of tongs, lateral view.
     C: Tongs in place as seen from above.

Risks. Excessive manipulation of the head-causing injury of the spinal cord during application is the major risk. Improper positioning of the tongs too high above the ears risks loss of hold in the bone and laceration of the scalp. Excessive anterior placement in the coronal plane causes an extension pull on the head and the risk of sudden violent extension if the patient is turned prone on the frame. Conversly, posterior placement causes a flexion force on the spine with the risk of further flexion when the patient is turned from the supine to the prone position.

Weight must be chosen carefully for the specific fracture and must seldom exceed 5 lbs for the upper cervical spine and 20 lbs for the lower cervical spine. Infection can occur about the pins, particularly with prolonged traction and as a result of poor pin care. Loosening of the device is seen more commonly in other types of tongs but still can occur in any device. Generally, it is associated with low grade infection and minimal motion of the metal tongs in the skull. Excessive pressure on the back of the head can produce occipital decubitus unless the patient is turned frequently and nursed carefully. The likelihood of this occipital decubitus is increased with anterior positioning of the tongs creating an extension force and increasing the pressure on the skin posteriorly.

Application Technique for Crutchfield Tongs. Crutchfield tongs are applied much in the same fashion as the Gardner tongs except that it is necessary to incise the skin and perforate the outer cortex of the skull with a specialized drill in order to secure their grip on the bone. In order to select the exact position before inserting the two points of the Crutchfield tongs, it is necessary to rotate the metal loop provided for the traction cord 180 degrees from its proper position for traction (Fig. 9). The span of the tongs is then adjusted until the two points touch the scalp in alignment with the axis of the cervical spine (Fig. 7). At the same time, the metal loop of the center portion of the tongs touches the scalp in the midsagittal plane. Once again, the ideal position is directly over the external auditory meatus. Obviously, Crutchfield tongs will not reach down to slightly above the ear as the Gardner tongs do.

Once the head is shaved and prepped locally, a small incision is placed where the two points indicate the ideal position. The galea is cleaned off a small area of bone and the drill hole is made in the outer table. Then, the metal loop is rotated back into its position for traction and the points of the tongs are placed deep within the holes. The locking nuts are tightened and the traction line is secured to the metal loop. It is not uncommon for the incisions in the scalp to produce a mild amount of bleeding, and a suture or two is occasionally required at the conclusion of the procedure. As with the Gardner tongs, it is important to slightly elevate the head end of the turning frame or bed on which the patient is lying to prevent the patient from

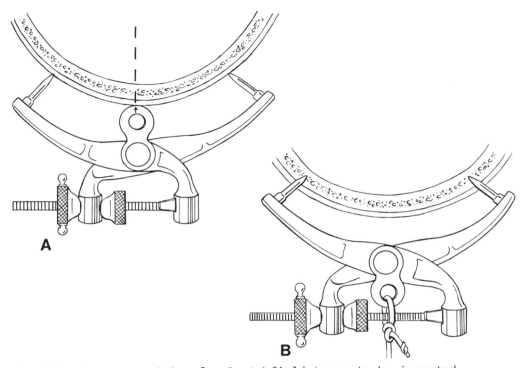

Fig. 9 A: Proper position for Crutchfield tongs to be inserted.
       B: Crutchfield tongs in place with loop now rotated to accept
            traction line.

gradually sliding toward the traction and eventually diminishing the
force of the pull. Most spinal frames are designed for this position.
If a hospital bed is being used, elevate the head end with shock blocks
and keep the patient's mattress flat otherwise the patient cannot be
turned easily.

     Risks. Potential problems anticipated for the Crutchfield tongs
are essentially the same as these risks described with Gardner-Wells
tongs.

Outpatient Head Halter Traction

     Indications. Intermittent cervical traction is advocated in the
treatment of neck pain redicular discomfort secondary to disc disease.

     Application. Generally, this form of traction is provided by com-
mercially available devices which clamp or hook over the top of a standard door.   The patient places the halter over the head with 1 pad beneath the chin and the other beneath the occiput. He then attaches this

to a spreader that is already tied to the traction line running over the pulley and ending in a water bag weight. The favored position is to sit facing the door which adds slight flexion to the traction force. Routines vary with treating orthopaedic surgeons, but generally the patient uses traction for a total of about 30 min. per day with weight varying from 10 to 20 lbs (Fig. 10).

Risks. Risks are few if patients are carefully instructed in the use of this device. The most common complaint is that the traction increases their pain. If this happens, the patient should be instructed to discontinue the traction until they consult their treating physician.

Halo Ring Traction

Indications. The halo ring provides an alternate means of skull traction for spinal injuries or spinal deformity. Compared to skull tongs, the direction of the traction force can be controlled more readily with the halo ring, and there is no movement between the skull and the fixation pins. The principle advantage of the halo ring is that it allows the patient out of bed while traction is maintained. Although initially introduced into Orthopaedics for use in cervical spine fractures, the halo has been used subsequently in the treatment of unstable thoracic spine fractures and to control or correct severe spinal deformities.

Application. There are five halo ring sizes, and the one chosen for a specific patient should allow approximately 1 to 1.5 cm clearance on all sides of the head. Each ring has numerous threaded holes for placement of three or four spacer discs to position the ring (Fig. 11A) and the four sterile pointed pins used for the skull fixation (Fig. 11B).

The halo ring may be applied on the day of injury or later as a substitute for initial head halter or skull tong traction. Head halter traction can be maintained during the halo ring application. An assistant gently lifts the head from the stretcher or supports the head off the end of the table to provide space for the ring to be positioned around the patient's head. Spacer pins and discs are applied to the central anterior halo ring hole and the two most posterior holes to give temporary fixation to the ring. This permits minor adjustments until the ideal position for the pins is obtained. Four fixation pins are used. The ring must be placed below the equator of the skull to prevent cephalad displacement.

Skin areas beneath the holes selected are swabbed with Betadine and sterile pins are inserted after 1% xylocaine has been injected into the skin, subcutaneous tissue, and scalp periosteum. The hair is generally not shaved. Two anterior pins are symmetrically placed in the frontal bone groove superior and lateral to the supraorbital ridge so that the ring margin lies about 1/2 cm above the lateral eyebrows. If the use

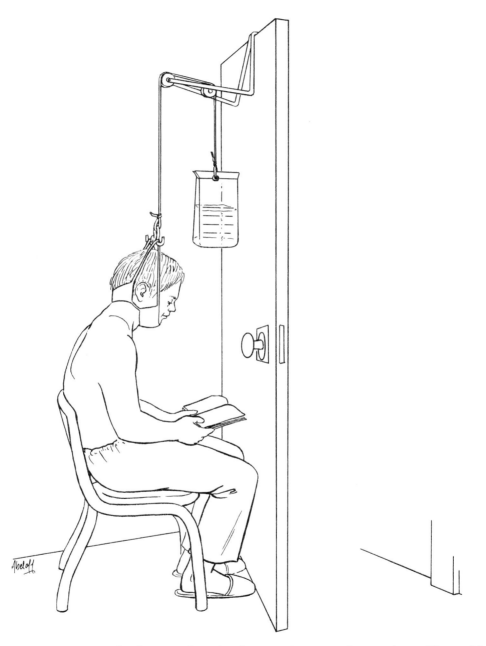

Fig. 10: Home cervical traction in its most commonly used configuration.

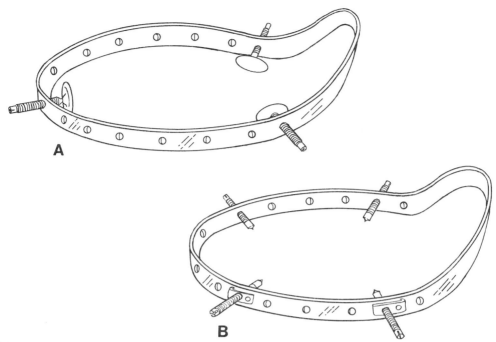

Fig. 11A: Halo ring with spacer pins.
Fig. 11B: Halo ring with skull fixation pins and locks.

of the halo is for a relatively short period of time, such as traction
for correction of spinal deformity, the anterior pins can be placed in
the hairline just posterior to the supraorbital ridge.

        Posteriorly, the pins are generally best positioned posterior and
superior to the external ear since the halo ring should be just above
the external ear. The halo must not touch the ear since it will aggra-
vate the patient who is unable to move away from the fixed ring. After
the ring has been properly positioned, and the proposed pin site cleaned and anesthetized, the sterile pins are inserted with finger pressure
until initial pin purchase is obtained. To keep the ring centered,
diagonally opposite pins should be tightened simultaneously (Fig. 12A).
After pins are finger-tight, the positioning discs are removed and the
final pin tightening is accomplished with torque screwdrivers. Generally 5 or 6 inch-pounds of pressure is ideal. Again, diagonally opposing
pins are tightened simultaneously. In small children with thin skulls,
3 or 4 inch-pounds of torque may be sufficient for fixation. Finally,
the set screws are tightened to lock the halo pins in place and prevent
loosening. At this point, it is possible to keep the patient in traction or to attach the halo ring to a plaster or plastic jacket.

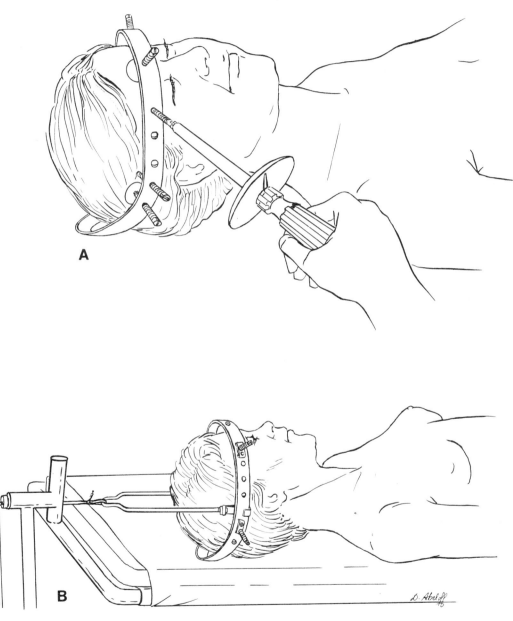

Fig. 12A: Corrective position of halo ring on patient's head.
Fig. 12B: Halo ring traction.

If traction is continued, appropriate flexion or extension forces, as indicated for the individual patient, may be obtained by placement of the traction pull more anteriorly for extension, or more posteriorly for flexion. The traction line can be attached directly to the halo ring with a Y-shaped rope or specially designed metal frame   (Fig. 12B). A headrest or skate attachment may also be applied to the ring decreasing direct ring pressure and allowing more free head movement. This will also prevent the pins from catching in the bedsheet. In the treatment of fractures, the amount of weight should not exceed the amount generally used with tong traction.

The major use of the halo ring is in combination with a body jacket to immobilize the cervical spine and allow the patient out of bed. If a plaster jacket is used, it is applied on a Risser frame with the head supported by an assistant to prevent neck movement. Careful molding over the iliac crest area is necessary to prevent the cast from slipping up or down. After the plaster cast is completed, the halo ring is attached to it by metallic uprights. The fixation is most secure if three uprights are used.

Before the halo ring is finally secured to these uprights, all connecting nuts and bolts are loosened and the surgeon positions the halo to obtain his desired cervical spine alignment. X-rays are obtained and minor adjustments are accomplished until the surgeon is satisfied with the position. The pins should be tightened to 6 inch-pounds of torque on one occasion during the first week the patient is in the device. They should not be tightened again.

Alternatively, the halo ring may be attached to a commercially available, sheepskin-lined, plastic body jacket with shoulder straps (Fig. 13). In patients with sensory loss over the trunk area, extreme care must be taken in plaster application, and the plastic body jacket is usually preferrable since it is possible to selectively loosen portions of the plastic jacket to check for skin pressure problems easily without disturbing alignment of the cervical spine. Once the halo brace or cast has been applied, the patient may sit or ambulate if his neurologic function and general health permit. X-rays are obtained after increased activity and if there is no evidence of change, the patient may be discharged in the halo cast or jacket.

Daily pin cleaning with antiseptic solution is the only other care required and this is usually accomplished by a family member. If pin is present at the pin site after the first few days, that pin has likely become loose and requires replacement in another halo pin hole. When one halo pin is being replaced, the other three will maintain sufficient fixation so that there is no loss of stability. Three months or more of halo wear is generally tolerated routinely. The removal of the halo pins and halo ring requires no local anesthesia and can be performed readily as an outpatient. Antiseptic solution applied to the wound for a few days following pin removal will generally allow rapid healing of

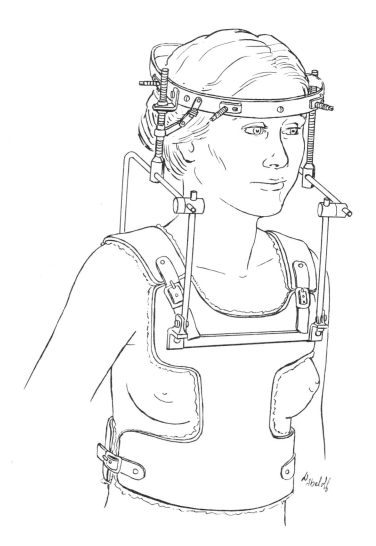

Fig. 13: Low profile halo with sheepskin lined plastic jacket.

the pin site.

When surgical decompression or fusion is indicated, placement of the patient in a halo jacket or a halo cast preoperatively lends greater safety when turning and positioning under general anesthesia. However, the halo may create some difficulty for the anesthetist and nasotracheal intubation is preferrable for patients in this unit.

Risks. The major risks of halo ring use are those also associated with skull tong placement. Inflammation around the pin sites, associated with purulent or seropurulent drainage should be cultured and treated with appropriate antibiotics. If drainage and inflammation persist or if pain worsens, infections of pin tracts must be treated with pin removal and reinsertion of a new pin in an adjacent area. If the pins have been removed and drainage persists, it may be necessary to curette that area of the skull to accomplish local debridement. This would usually be accompanied by appropriate antibiotic therapy.

Penetration of the pins through both bony tables can produce a cerebrospinal fluid leak. The treatment is removal of the pin and antibiotic therapy to prevent meningitis. Such a cerebrospinal fluid leak will generally seal spontaneously and intradural abscesses are very rare. Attempts to radiographically visualize a penetrated halo pin are difficult and rely on x-rays of each single pin tangential to the skull at the site of entry of the pin. These films are not routinely done and may convey a false impression of safety unless the exact angle is obtained. If penetration is suspected, it is best to immediately change the pin.

Scars over the eyebrows are objectionable to some and necessitate need for plastic surgical revision. Slippage of the head ring can lacerate the scalp but this can be avoided if the ring is placed below the equator of the skull. Pressure sores may develop beneath a cast, particularly in a neurologically impaired patient who is insensate over the trunk region.

The halo ring has opened a new dimension to treatment of cervical spine injuries permitting safe nursing and ambulation of the seriously injured. If used properly, it facilitates rehabilitation, cuts hospital costs, and provides excellent stability. Because of the efficiency of this method, however, there is a tendency to overuse the halo ring. It should be reserved for unstable spine fractures and not used when lesser neck bracing methods will suffice.

TRACTION FOR SPINAL DEFORMITY

The treatment of spinal deformity frequently includes the use of traction, either diagnostically or as a vital part of the operative method. Traction is unnecessary for the usual operative treatment of idiopathic scoliosis and is contraindicated in patients with spastic cerebral palsy or myelomeningocele.

The main traction used for spinal deformity is that associated with the use of a halo ring, but one non-invasive technique used in some centers is that device by Cotrel of France.

Indications: Cotrel Traction. Cotrel traction has been utilized preoperatively in an attempt to improve intra-operative corrections, although there is disagreement as to its efficacy. In addition, Cotrel himself uses this traction in place of bracing for idiopathic scoliosis, but this approach has not been successfully duplicated in the United States. The principle feature of this traction is its dynamic nature which allows the patient to participate actively in correction of the spinal deformity.

Another use of Cotrel traction is in older scoliosis patients with marked curvatures and low back pain. The Cotrel traction unit can be adapted to use at home during periods of increased symptoms. This approach has been useful in avoiding surgery in some older patients.

Application. Units of Cotrel traction are commercially available in the United States. They include a head halter and pelvic band connected by a variety of pulleys and ropes (Fig. 14A). Once assembled, the patient extends his hips and knees pushing the foot pieces distally. This force is transmitted to the head halter straightening the spine while the pelvic band stabilizes the pelvis (Fig. 14B). The net result is longitudinal traction. It is possible to adjust the amount of tension on these ropes and pulleys. Cotrel claims that with this apparatus normal people can generate 30 to 40 kg of force.

The dynamic traction is used for at least two periods of therapy each day, and the patient sleeps in a static traction unit using the same head halter and pelvic band arrangement. Static traction of more than 15 lbs is not well tolerated and a traction angle of greater than 40 degrees from the horizontal puts excessive pressure on the chin. If Cotrel traction is used preoperatively, it is possible to determine the flexibility of a spinal deformity. The correction obtained with Cotrel traction is very comparable to the actual correction obtained with Harrington rod instrumentation and fusion.

Risks. With the Cotrel traction, there are virtually no complications of note. During the time that traction is applied, it is difficult to talk or eat. A bite block may be necessary if pain develops in the temporomandibular joints. Long term or prolonged use of the head halter has, in Cotrel's experience, led to occasional orthodontic or mandibular abnormalities.

Indications: Halo Femoral Traction. This traction is used as an aid in the correction of severe spinal deformities and occasionally in combination with spinal osteotomy as the first part of a staged correc-

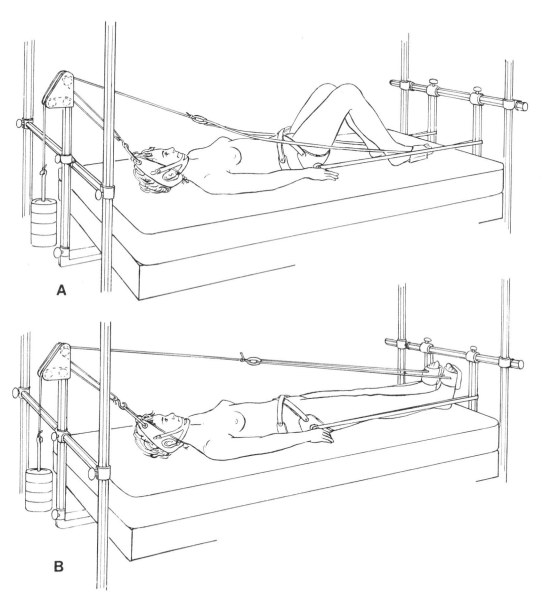

Fig.   14A: Cotrel traction in relaxed position.
Fig.   14B: Cotrel traction in extended position.

tion.

Application. Under general anesthesia, the halo is positioned as previously described and distal femoral traction is applied with Steinmann pins or Kirschner wires. After positioning the halo ring and femoral pins, the patient is nursed on a Stryker frame (Fig. 15) while traction force weight is gradually increased over a 7 to 14 day period. Initial weights range from 5 or 10 lbs at each end with a maximum limit of one-third to one-half the patient's weight.

Daily neurological examinations are performed and any neurologic abnormality is treated at once by decreasing the weights and observing the patient for the recovery of the neurologic deficit. The principle examination involves the cranial nerves (particularly, the VI, IX, X, and XII),reflexes, strength and sensation of upper and lower limbs, and bladder function. Lateral rectus muscle palsy from the compression of the VI cranial nerve and increasing hyperreflexia or clonus of the lower extremities are the most common abnormalities seen as signs of impending neurologic loss.

When treating spinal deformities with the halo femoral traction, no further correction is generally seen after 2 weeks. When maximum benefit has been obtained, surgery to maintain this correction is accomplished by Harrington rod instrumentation and spinal fusion. The traction remains in place during the surgery. The halo and pins are removed postoperatively, while the patient is under anesthesia, and the remainder of the care is routine.

Occasionally, it is not possible to firmly secure the Harrington instrumentation. When this occurs, the surgeon may elect to leave the halo on and attach this through rigid uprights to a plaster body jacket or plastic pelvic mold to maintain the traction force in the postoperative period (Fig. 16). This same device can also be used to stabilize a thoracic spinal fracture preventing further kyphos as it heals.

Risks. Major complications from halo femoral traction are the neurologic difficulties mentioned above. Problems associated with the halo pins and femoral pins are generally minor although transient knee stiffness may persist after femoral pin removal.

Halo Pelvic Apparatus

Indications. The halo pelvic apparatus is most commonly used to treat patients with severe spinal deformities from tuberculosis or polio. The device consists of a halo and large metal hoop anchored to the pelvis by pins passing through each iliac.

Application. The application of the halo has been discussed previously in this chapter. The pelvic ring is applied under general anes-

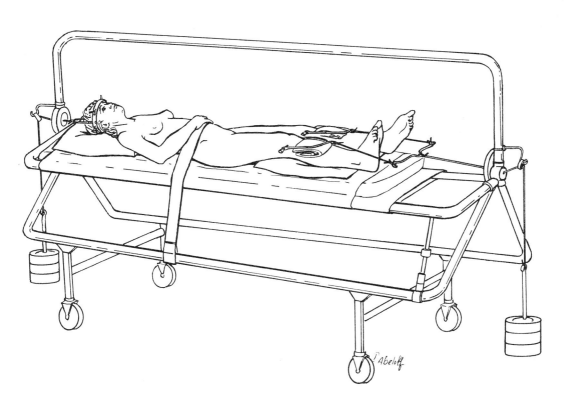

Fig. 15:   Halo Femoral Traction.

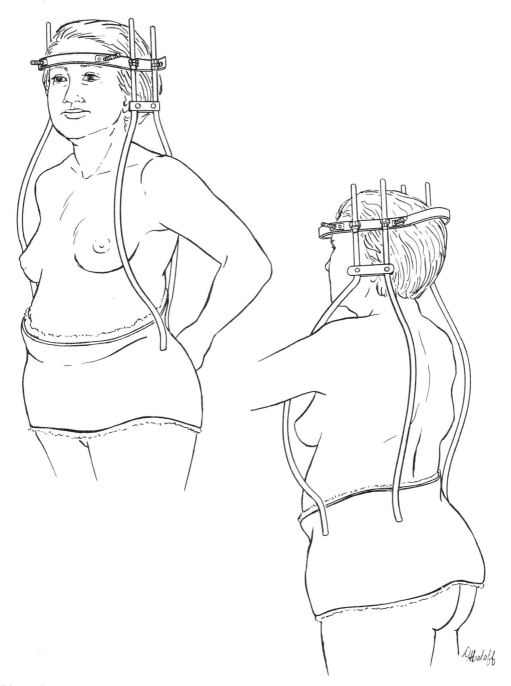

Fig. 16:   Halo ring in conjunction with pelvic girdle for thoracic
           and lumbar spine deformity or injury.

thesia. The patient is positioned laterally while the iliac pin is
placed in the opposite or "up" side. After the initial pelvic pin has
been placed, the patient is turned 180 degrees, again positioned laterally, and the other iliac pin is placed. The lateral positioning is
necessary to allow the intestines to drop away from the area of pin insertion. Although a jig is available, the author prefers use of a small
incision anteriorly placing these pins under direct vision. The pelvic
pin enters approximately 3 cm behind the anterosuperior iliac spine in
the area of relative bony thickness. This pin is directed posteriorly
and medially to exit just lateral to the posterior iliac spine. With
the author's technique, the surgeon can observe the pin as it passes
through the iliac fossa and be certain that no damage is done in case
the pin comes out of the bone in the mid portion of the ilium. Iliac
crest bone graft is often obtained at this time and stored for later use
during spinal fusion.

After insertion of the pins, the pelvic hoop is attached. It is
necessary to allow at least 2.5 cm clearance on each side of the pelvis.
Four rigid uprights with turnbuckles connect the pelvic hoop to the halo
ring (Fig. 17). Gradual lengthening is carried out to slowly correct
the rigid spinal deformity.

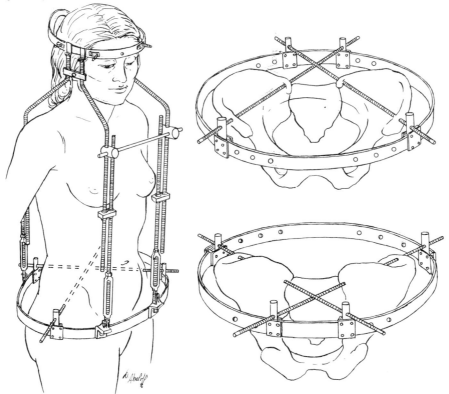

Fig. 17: Halo pelvic traction.

Risks. Although this device is rigid and effective, there are a
large number of possible complications because of the fixed traction
force. First, the incidence of spinal cord injury with resultant neurologic deficit is higher with this form of treatment than any other type
of halo traction. If a deficit is seen during the daily neurologic examination, tension on the uprights should be reduced immediately. Second, long term use of halo pelvic traction has lead to degenerative
changes of the cervical spine and prolonged excessive traction has been
blamed for aseptic necrosis of the odontoid. Third, drainage from the
pelvic pins is a fairly common occurrence because of fatty tissue in the
area of the iliac crest. If these pins subsequently become infected,
loosening may result and replacement of these pelvic pins is difficult
in the face of infection. Four, if spinal surgery is to be performed,
the use of pelvic pins increases the difficulty obtaining iliac crest
bone graft and limits the amount of bone graft that can be used.

Because of the increased risk of neurologic injury, the halo pelvic
apparatus remains a technique to be used principally where other techniques are not applicable.

Halo Suspension Traction

Indications. Because of the possible neurologic problems inherent
in the fixed type of traction (halo, pelvic), halo suspension traction
as advocated by Stagnara of Lyon, France, has some appeal. This traction is generally used preoperatively either to obtain gradual correction of the deformity or to maintain position following first stage
osteotomies. It is typically employed for a 1- to 3-week period prior to
definitive instrumentation and fusion. Halo suspension eliminates the
need for continuous immobilization in bed and may diminish some of the
otherwise numerous postoperative problems that develop as a result of
prolonged bed rest. It is expected that this method of traction will
increase in popularity over the next few years.

Application. The halo ring is applied in a standard fashion. After
halo application, force is exerted by using the patient's own weight as
a countertraction. He is then managed in a specially designed wheelchair with an overhead pulley frame during the day (Fig. 18A), and an
inclined bed at night (Fig. 18B). Weights on the halo ring are gradually increased to one-third or one-half body weight, as with other halo
traction techniques for severe spinal deformity.

Risks. The potential complications or risks are essentially those of
other skeletal spinal traction and daily neurologic examinations are
essential. However, fixed traction is not being applied from both ends
simultaneously in this situation so the potential neurologic deficit is
diminished to some degree.

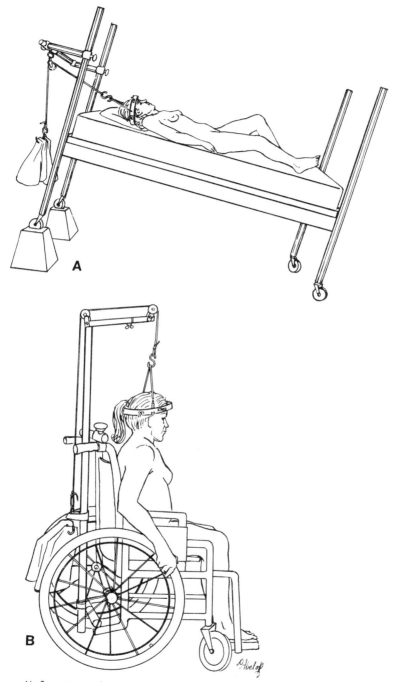

Fig. 18A : Halo traction in wheelchair.
Fig. 18B : Nighttime halo suspension on incline bed.

LUMBAR TRACTION

Inpatient Pelvic Belt Traction

Indications. Pelvic belt traction is indicated for the conservative treatment of low back pain or for the initial care of a suspected lumbar disc herniation. This traction is generally not indicated for the treatment of pelvic or lumbar spine fractures. It has 2 advantages over bilateral bucks treatment. First, the patient is able to apply or discontinue the traction without assistance. Second, higher weights can be loterated with the pelvic belt.

Application. The patient is placed supine in the bed and the belt device is either wrapped or secured with buckles or velcro fastening (Fig. 19). It is important that the belt is around the pelvis, not squeezing or gripping the patient above the level of the iliac crest. The weight loops provided on either side of the belt receive the traction line which leads through pulleys at the foot of the bed to the weight carriers. Initially, 5 lbs are placed on each side. This can be increased gradually to a maximum of 15 lbs on each line for a total of 30 lbs of pelvic traction. The patient is best positioned in semi-Fowler's position, the head of the bed slightly keeps the patient from sliding down when the heavier weights are used.

Risks. The risks of traction of this type are minimal except for excessive weights which can cause skin problems and discomfort over the superior portion of the iliac crest.

Home Pelvic Traction

Indications. Intermittent home pelvic traction is indicated in the conservative treatment of low back pain or in the initial evaluation of the suspected herniated disc. It is especially useful because the patient can readily apply and remove this traction belt. The entire setup is simple and can be used in the patient's bed at home.

Application. The patient lies supine with a pillow beneath the head and knees. The pelvic device is secured either with buckles or velcro depending on the type available. Prior to setting up the traction, bedboards must be placed beneath the mattress to stiffen the surface on which he will be lying. Once applied, traction lines are led through the weight loops and down over the foot of the bed. At this point, the pulley system becomes quite variable. If the bed has a footboard, standard pulleys can be attached to this and weights led over the end. Otherwise, it is necessary to use a device such as a sawhorse or small table that can brace itself against the bottom of the bed. Be aware that excessive weight will cause him to slide toward the bottom of the bed. If this becomes a problem, small shock blocks or bricks can be placed under the foot of the bed (Fig. 20).

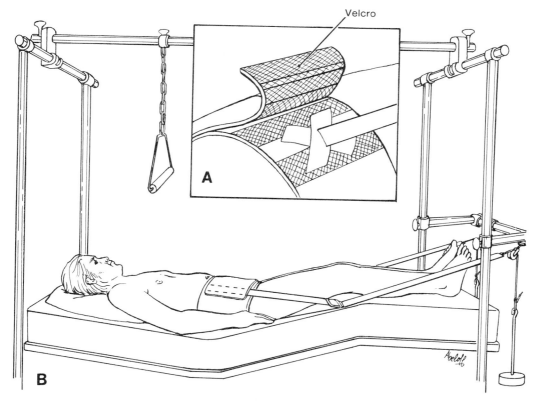

Velcro

A

B

Fig. 19: Inpatient pelvic belt traction.

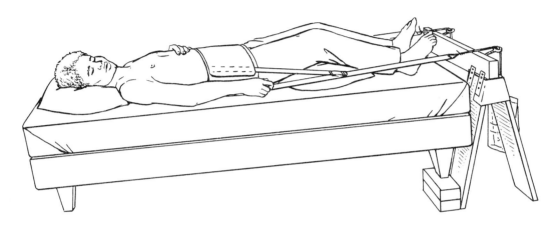

Fig. 20 :   Home pelvic traction.

* * * * * * * * *

   Risks. The risks to the patient are minimal if the technique and system is carefully explained. The back pain can be aggravated by traction and if this happens, the patient should be instructed to discontinue the traction and contact their physician for further instructions.

REFERENCES

1. Barton, L.G.: The Reduction of Fracture Dislocation of the Cervical
        Vertebrae by Skeletal Traction; Surg. Gyn. and Obst.,
        67:94, 1938.

2. Crutchfield, W.G.: Skeletal Traction in the Treatment of Injuries
        to the Cervical Spine; J.A.M.A., 155:29, 1954.

3. Crutchfield, W.G.: Treatment of Injuries of the Cervical Spine;
        J.B.J.S., 20:696, 1938.

4. Evans, D.K.: Reduction of Cervical Dislocation; J.B.J.S., 43B:552,
        1961.

5. Gallie, W.E.: Skeletal Traction in the Treatment of Fractures and
        Dislocations of the Cervical Spine; Annals of Surg.,
        Oct.:770, 1937.

6. Goldie, I.F.: The Biomechanical Influence of Traction on the Cer-
        vical Spine; Scand. J. Rehab. Med., 9:31, 1977.

7. Harris, P.R.: Cervical Traction: Review of the Literature and
        Treatment Guidelines; Physical Therapy, 57:910, 1977.

8. Judovich, B.D.: Herniated Cervical Disc: A New Form of Traction
        Therapy; Amer. J. Surg., Dec.:646, 1952.

9. Laurin, C.A.: Cervical Traction in the Home; Beneral Practice,
        94:36, 1966.

10. Loeser, J.D.: History of Skeletal Traction in the Treatment of
        Cervical Spine Injuries; J. Neurosurg., 33:54, 1970.

11. Norton, W.L.: Fractures and Dislocations of the Cervical Spine;
        J.B.J.S., 44A:115, 1962.

12. Rockwood, C.A.: Fractures; J.B. Lippincott Co., Philadelphia, 1975.

13. Valtonen, E.J.: Cervical Traction as a Therapeutic Tool; Scan. J.
        Rehab. Med., 2:29, 1970.

14. Vinke, T.H.: A Skull-Traction Apparatus; J.B.J.S., 30A:522, 1948.

15. Mathews, J.A.: Lumbar Traction: A Double-Blind Controlled Study
        for Sciatica; Rheumatology and Rehab., 14:222, 1975.

CHAPTER 4

Upper Extremity Traction

Most fractures of the clavicle, shoulder, humeral shaft, and elbow can be managed in traction. This implies that the patient must be at bed rest. Because orthopaedic surgeons have developed techniques over the years to treat simple fractures of the upper extremity keeping the patient ambulatory, traction is commonly reserved for the multiply injured or comatose individual with complicated fractures where hospitalization and bed rest are essential.

Both skin traction and skeletal traction are used in the upper extremity. The former is employed more commonly when the weight required is minimal and traction is more of a stabilizing or elevating device. The latter skeletal traction is used more often for the difficult fractures in or about the elbow, since forces far in excess of that tolerated by the patient's skin may be required.

Skin Traction. Skin traction is achieved by attaching various types of adhesive strips over large areas of an extremity. It generally will withstand a traction force of up to 10 lbs for about 4 weeks without slipping. This form of traction is particularly suitable for younger children because of their fast healing and the lighter forces required for reduction and immobilization. Furthermore, skin traction does not expose the bone to possible infection or risk damage to the epiphyseal growth apparatus.

There are, of course, disadvantages to skin traction. Most young patients and some older ones exhibit the unfortunate tendency to disarrange the elastic bandage or tunnel their fingers under the traction tape. Skin traction cannot be used to control rotation. It cannot withstand the magnitude and duration of forces required for larger bones of adults, and it should never be applied to injured skin.

Simple Forearm Skin Traction (Fig. 21)

Indications. This type of traction has two major functions. First, it is most useful for elevation in any upper extremity injury, particularly in the comatose or unreliable patient who is uncooperative. It is ideal for the patient who cannot tolerate a hand resting on their chest such as a patient with extensive wounds, burns, or chest tubes. Forearm skin traction is excellent treatment for the difficult clavicle fracture. Most of these reduce easily with the patient supine. The arm is supported in slight abduction with the elbow mildly flexed. This method has been named the "beauty queen" approach to clavicle fractures and is

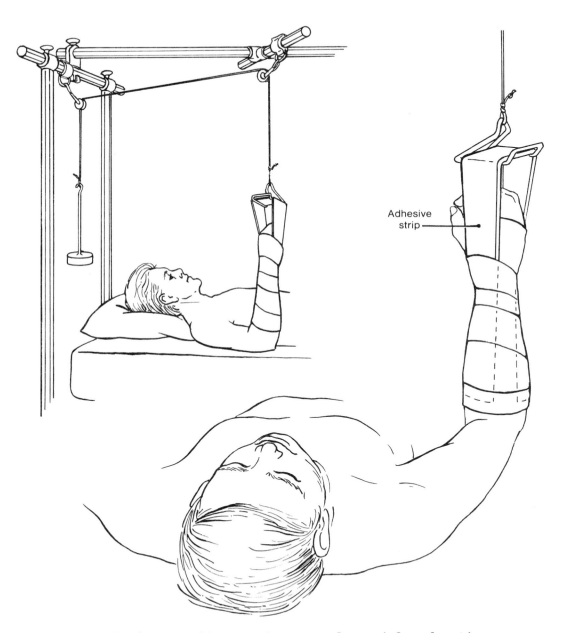

Adhesive
strip

Fig. 21: Simple forearm skin traction commonly used for elevation.

said to produce excellent cosmetic results after several weeks of bed rest.

Application. The patient is placed supine at bed rest. After several layers of protective soft roll are placed over the bony prominences at the wrist, the adhesive strip is applied. These strips can be either commercially available sponged material with gummed backing or plain adhesive tape. Paper tape should never be used. If the traction is to be on for some time, it is prudent to shave and prep the forearm before application of the adhesive strips. The strips are applied down one side of the forearm and looped over the hand leaving sufficient room for full extension of the fingers. The second arm of the loop is then applied to the opposite side of the forearm and the ace bandage is wrapped snuggly over the adhesive strip. The purpose of the ace bandage is to make a more even contact for the adhesive material and to provide a better hold. If the ace bandage is wrapped too tightly, however, edema can develop in the hand. This must be checked frequently during the first 24 hrs.

Generally, the long gummed strips or pieces of adhesive tape are used in this loop fashion; however, it is possible to use multiple adhesive strips and join them over the fingers, taping them directly to a traction yoke. If the yoke is not available, a simple block of wood through which traction can be applied is acceptable (Fig. 22).

A clavicle fracture is treated with the arm abducted 30 degrees from the body, and the elbow flexed approximately 30 degrees. The traction line is then run through a pulley attached to an outrigger from the fracture bed and 4 to 5 lbs of traction is applied. The patient must remain supine with only a pillow beneath the head.

When elevation is the goal, the same line is attached directly over the elbow so that the elbow itself is flexed 90 degrees and the forearm is vertical directly in line with the traction pull. A comfortable amount of shoulder abduction is permitted in this circumstance and the head of the bed may be raised for meals, etc.

Risks. The major risk in this type of traction is skin loss which can be caused by excessive weight generally above 7 to 10 lbs. Too much weight can create a sheer force along the skin line and result in severe blistering with second degree skin loss beneath the adhesive strips. Secondly, traction in combination with excessive abduction of the shoulder can compromise the subclavian vessels or produce a painful impingement of the rotator cuff between the lateral acromion and the greater tuberosity. Third, overly tight wrapping of the forearm can create circulatory embarrassment to the fingers. In this same sense, swelling from the injury can lead to circulatory embarrassment and can only be avoided by frequent checks of the injured extremity in traction.

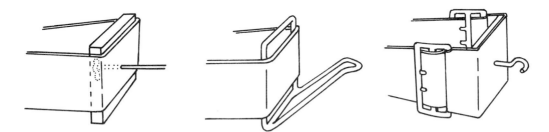

Fig. 22: Several yokes available to receive the adhesive strips used
         for any skin traction.

Double Skin Traction: Forearm and Upper Arm (Fig.23)

Indications. This form of traction is most useful in the treatment
of greater tuberosity or proximal humeral shaft fractures in the multiply injured patient already restricted to bed. As simple forearm skin
traction, it can be used for the conservative care of clavicle fracture
and may be more comfortable for the patient because of the 90 degrees
flexion of the elbow.

Application. The patient is placed supine, and in the same fashion
as previously described, the forearm adhesive strips are placed. The
yoke is attached to an overhead pulley and the arm abducted 30 degrees,
the elbow flexed 90 degrees. The second component of this traction is
applied with the adhesive strip and ace bandage to the upper arm. This
extends from approximately the junction of the middle third of the humerus, while the overhead line can alter both elbow flexion and humeral
rotation depending on where the overhead pulley is located.

Risks. Excessive weight of more than 7 to 10 lbs on the forearm
component and of 5 to 7 lbs on the upper arm component can cause second
degree skin loss beneath the adhesive strips. Too much weight on the
upper arm portion of this traction can lead to slippage of the entire
bandage causing it to act like a tourniquet around the antecubital

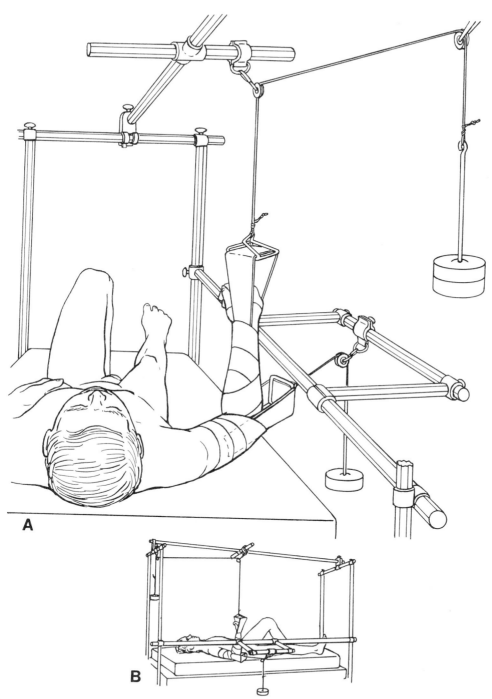

Fig. 23: Double skin traction - forearm and upper arm.

space. Tight wrapping of the upper arm bandage can also lead to edema
in the antecubital and elbow area. A combination of tight wrap and too
much weight can be very treacherous causing sufficient construction
around the elbow to produce forearm ischemia. Finally, an active patient will have difficulty tolerating this traction. They find them-
selves drifting toward the traction forces and respond to this by moving about in bed risking angulation of their fracture. It is generally
advised that when the patient is mobile enough to engage in this activity, that they are better treated with Velpeau dressing or a long arm
cast.

Dunlop's Traction

Indications. Dunlop's traction is used for the treatment of supracondylar and transcondylar fractures in children. It is generally
limited to the fracture which does not lend itself easily to closed reduction or a clinical setting where elbow flexion is likely to compromise circulation. With the gentle pull provided in this traction
arrangement, an acceptable reduction is usually obtained and the patient held until the swelling subsides. After approximately 10 days,
a long arm cast is applied for the duration of treatment and the patient is discharged.

A second indication of Dunlop's traction is following a difficult
or traumatic closed reduction. The traction will then function to hold
the reduction and provide easy access to the arm for evaluating the
circulation.

Application. The patient is placed supine in the hospital bed or
crib with the affected arm extending out from the bed (Fig. 24). It is
often necessary to use either the crib side or bed rail to prevent the
patient from slipping too far over the side of the bed. When this is
done, there should be some padding placed between the patient and these
hard restraints. The sides are secured so that they are not accident-
ally dropped or lowered on to the injured extremity.

The forearm skin traction is applied in a standard way leaving a
large loop over the fingers. The arm is then moderately abducted and
the traction line attached to the yoke beneath the adhesive strip looped
over the hand. This is carried through a pulley to an outrigger and a
light weight is applied. Next, a padded sling is constructed out of
heavy felt and wrapped over the distal humerus. Through a hole in the
felt, a weight is attached. The extremity is then balanced in the
traction so that the arm remains comfortably abducted and the elbow
flexed. The humeral shaft should be slightly elevated from the edge of
the bed by the traction, and the elbow should be positioned at approximately 135 degrees of flexion.

Occasionally, it is necessary to elevate the same side of the bed
on small shock blocks to counter the traction weights tending to pull

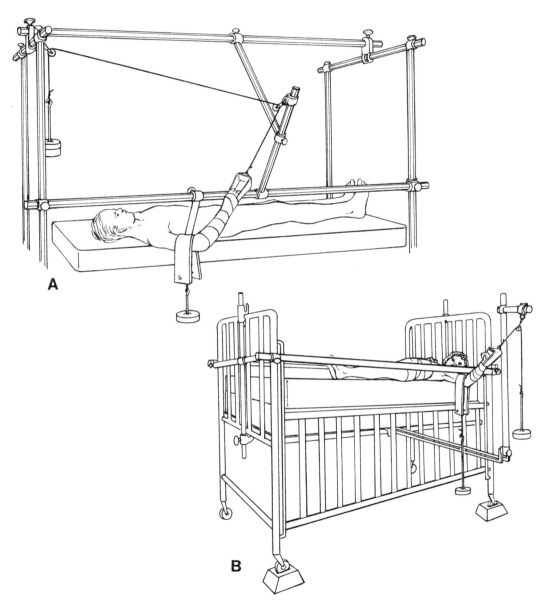

Fig. 24A: Dunlop's skin traction for the larger child in a fracture bed.
      24B: Dunlop's traction for a child in a crib.

the patient toward the side of the bed.

The weights required for the forearm and humeral aspects of this traction vary considerably. In the smaller child, often the weight hanger alone is sufficient for the humeral component while 1 to 2 lbs may be adequate for the forearm component. As a rule of thumb, start with lighter weights or weight sufficient to maintain the postion and very gradually add additional weight to the humeral component checking each increment with x-rays and observing the circulation. Over 24 hrs, it will be possible to obtain an adequate reduction and generally determine the minimum amount of weight required to hold this position.

Risks. The possibility of ischemic (or Volkmann's) contracture is the major concern in any transcondylar or supracondylar fracture. The circulatory state of the hand must be watched hourly for the first 10 to 12 hrs. Any indication of ischemia or elevated compartment pressures require immediate adjustment of the traction and reassessment of the bony alignment. If simple adjustment of the traction does not provide the necessary relief, further attempts at closed reduction, exploration of the artery, or even forearm fasciotomy must be considered.

Too much weight, particularly in the humeral portion of this traction, can lead to excessive edema of the elbow. This is frequently worrisome but soft dependent edema about the olecranon process is seldom significant and does not generally alter the patient's final result.

Finally, there is considerable risk to the arm itself since it is protruding from the side of the bed. Visitors and nursing personnel must be constantly aware of the risk to this extremity as they move about the bed.

Olecranon Pin Traction (Overhead)

Indications. Olecranon pin traction has enjoyed considerable popularity and generally replaced Dunlop's traction in many centers as a standard method for treating difficult supracondylar fractures (Fig. 25). It is also useful for the treatment of comminuted or open fractures of the distal humerus, but more proximal injuries tend to be displaced by this overhead position and are generally not managed in this fashion.

Its advantages are several. First, it provides rigid skeletal fixation for traction forces greater than that capable with skin techniques. Second, by moving the arm sling cephalad or caudad, but leaving the olecranon pin traction line in place, rotational correction can be affected. Third, changing a K-wire angle or moving the traction rope attached to the K-wire spreader bar will produce some angular correction. Fourth, it provides considerable elevation with the extremity directly above the heart. Fifth, the arm is confined within the protective enclosure of the bed and is less likely to be injured than with Dunlop's traction. Finally, the patient is able to gradually or partial-

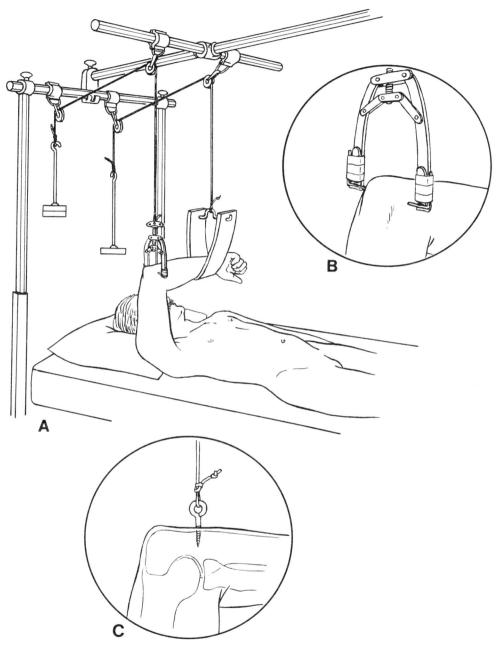

Fig. 25: Overhead olecran pin traction detail of upper insert shows
          the K-wire bent and taped over the outside of the traction
          bow. Lower insert, an alternative to the K-wire is an islet
          screw inserted at exactly the same point on the olecranon as
          the K-wire.

ly elevate the head of the bed after his fracture begins to heal.

Application. The patient is placed supine and the area of the proximal ulna prepped. The ideal position for insertion of the ulna K-wire
or screw in the average adult is approximately 1¼ inches distal to the
tip of the olecranon. It is important to place this fixation sufficiently distal to avoid the joint. On x-ray, the pin is well positioned
and it lies just distal to the coronoid process (Fig. 25).

The assistant supports the forearm with the upper arm slightly abducted away from the body. A moderate size K-wire is placed through
the proximal ulna. During application, the assistant provides the necessary pressure. The pin is passed with either a power K-wire inserter
or large hand drill. Generally, the surgeon has more room to approach
the bone in the proximal ulna when he works from the lateral aspect of
the ulna passing the pin medially. In this case, extreme care must be
taken to avoid injury to the ulnar nerve. Once the wire is through, a
traction bow is attached and gentle pull is exerted on the bone. The
forearm is then carried up and across the chest so that the humerus
points directly up, and the forearm lies approximately parallel with
the horizon. Next, the assistant supports the forearm while the surgeon attaches the traction line to an overhead pulley placed directly
above the patient's affected shoulder creating an imaginary straight
line between the patient's shoulder, elbow, and pulley overhead. Weight
is then applied, initially between 2 and 5 lbs.

With the assistant supporting the elbow, a felt sling covered with
stockinette is slipped over the forearm and a 6-inch spreader bar is
attached to a pulley placed directly over the patient's chest. A weight
of 1 to 2 lbs is generally adequate for this portion of the system initially. The support is released and the system balanced so that the
patient lies comfortably with the arm straight and the elbow flexed at
90 degrees. No shock blocks or restraints are required.

The weights must be balanced to keep the fracture well aligned and
only x-ray evaluation will provide this exacting information.

Risks. The risks of overhead olecranon pin traction are essentially
those associated with the fractures it is used to treat. There must be
constant vigilance for circulatory embarrassment to avoid ischemic
change or obstruction of venous outflow and subsequent compartment syndromes.

Excessive weight will lead to distraction of the fragments. Inadequate weight will allow them to angulate. Pin tract infection is a
possibility and careful, meticulous care is essential.

Occasionally, inadequate pin placement can lead the surgeon to be-
lieve the pin is in the ulna when in fact it is placed just subperi-
osteal over the bone. When weight is applied, the pin will gradually

cut out of the periosteum. This produces sharp pain and a sudden deformity puckering the skin. If such a problem develops, the pin is
simply removed under local anesthesia and a new olecranon transfixion
pin placed through the bone. Finally, ulnar nerve injury can result
from careless pin insertion.

Lateral Olecranon Pin Traction

Indications. This lateral skeletal traction can be used for any
humeral fracture much as double skin traction, except that higher forces
may be exerted on the fracture through the skeletal pin (Fig. 26). This
lateral position works well for the multiply injured or comatose patient
but is a very difficult traction to maintain in the alert, active person,
since they constantly slide toward the traction and move about the bed
risking angulation of their fracture.

Application. The ulnar pin is inserted as described previously and
the traction pull is applied to the K-wire or screw. The olecranon
traction line is then run from this bow through a lateral pulley. With
the arm in moderate abduction, a light traction weight is applied to
the olecranon line. This traction must be parallel with the imaginary
line of the bed for if it is below this line, there is a tendency to
pull the elbow down into the mattress causing a pressure sore over the
olecranon. If it is too high, it will flex the distal humerus causing
displacement or angulation of the fracture.

Next, the elbow is flexed to approximately 90 degrees, and skin traction is applied to the forearm after the ulnar styloid area has been
padded with soft roll. The traction line is run from the yoke through
a pulley placed directly over the patient's elbow and a 1- or 2 lb weight
is attached to this line. The patient and his extremity are protected
throughout this procedure by an assistant and only at this point is it
possible to gradually release the support and balance the traction lines
by adjusting the weights until the desired alignment is obtained.

When using forearm skin traction in combination with an olecranon pin,
the same weight limits previously described apply for the skin traction
portion of the setup. Generally, only minimal weight is required to
keep the elbow flexed to 90 degrees. The weight applied to the skeletal
pin or screw is generally larger. It is wise to start with 3 to 4 lbs
and increase gradually following the x-rays and clinical appearance of
the arm.

Risks. Excessive weight on the olecranon pin will distract the fracture and risk vascular embarrassment to the forearm. Inadequate weight
will allow angulation and shortening of the fracture. Improper placement of the overhead pulley will impart undesirable rotation to the humeral fracture and may lead to malunions. As with all varieties of
skeletal traction, pin care is important and improper or shallow pin
placement can allow the pin to cut out.

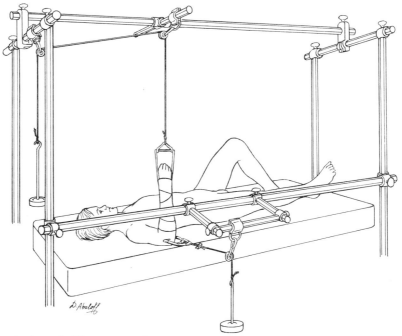

Fig. 26:   Lateral Olecranon Pin Traction (shown with K-wire and bow).

Metacarpal Pin Traction

    Indications. Metacarpal K-wire traction is most commonly used as
a method of obtaining and holding a difficult reduction, such as a
comminuted fracture of the distal radius. The pin can be used alone or
in combination with an upper arm sling or olecranon pin counterweights.
Once reduction is obtained, both metacarpal and olecranon pins are frequently incorporated in the cast. If it is not desirable to use a cast
immediately, these two pins can be attached to weighted lines and balanced traction employed (Fig. 27D). This provides a period of elevation
and observation, while alignment and length are preserved. It is an
especially useful method following a compound fracture requiring frequent dressing changes or for the first few days of treatment after a
difficult closed reduction.

    When the physician is faced with a patient whose extremity contains
several fractures such as combined humeral shaft and both bones of the
forearm, the metacarpal pin is very useful in maintaining traction of
the forearm in combination with olecranon pin traction to maintain
alignment of the humeral fracture. This arrangement lends itself to
delayed cast application with incorporation of the pins directly into
the plaster.

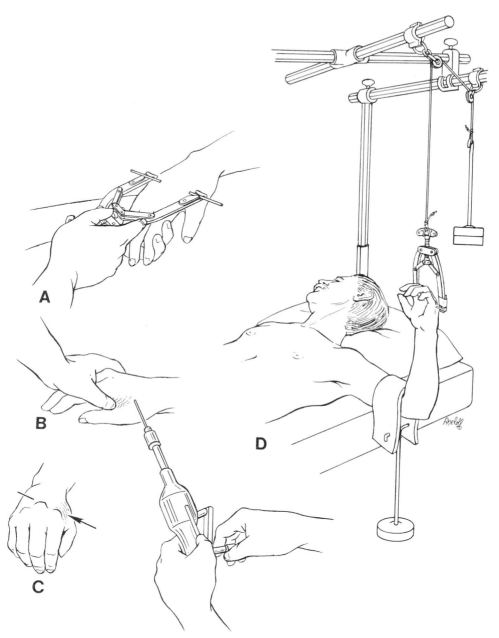

Fig. 27 : Balanced metacarpal pin traction with a sling counterweight.
A: Ideal pin placement in the proximal 2nd and 3rd metacarpals.
B: Technique of pin insertion with the assistant supporting the arched metacarpals.
C: Attaching the traction bow.

Application. The patient lies supine on the stretcher with the elbow flexed at 90 degrees, and the fingers are held by an assistant. The surgeon preps the metacarpal area generally at the proximal third of the second and third metacarpal. The hand is grasped and squeezed transversely so as to maximize the transverse arch of the metacarpals (Fig. 27 A). Beginning on the radial side of the hand, the K-wire is then inserted in the proximal portion of the second and third metacarpals (Fig. 27 B). Generally, it is not desirable to include the fourth metacarpal. With experience, this becomes a relatively easy procedure.

It is often possible for the surgeon to anticipate a required radial or ulnar angulation and he may place the pin in such a fashion that traction will tend to impart either radial or ulnar deviation to the fracture fragments. If necessary, an olecranon pin can then be inserted at the same time by prepping the area beneath the coronoid process and using the technique previously described.

The next step is to attach the traction bow to the metacarpal pin (Fig. 27 C). From this, a traction line runs straight up through a pulley placed directly above the patient's injured elbow. Once this has been accomplished and several pounds of weight are applied, the felt sling or olecranon pin counterweight is applied. If the olecranon pin is to provide countertraction, the weight hanger is suspended directly from its traction bow. Once the entire apparatus is assembled, support is gradually withdrawn from the forearm and fingers as the weights are balanced. X-rays are easily obtained to follow the position of the fracture and amount of weight required.

Risks. The risks of metacarpal pin traction are essentially those of any previously described in skeletal traction; infection, loosening, or improper positioning of the pin are all concerns. Specifically, the surgeon must use a moderately heavy pin if he plans to incorporate this into a cast later on or bending will occur allowing the fracture to shorten. Finally, stiffness of the intrinsic muscles is common after metacarpal pins and early active range of motion work of the fingers is essential.

Finger Trap Traction

Indications. Chinese finger traps have been a favorite device of the orthopaedic resident for many years. They are utilized to hold the patient's hand elevated and assist in reduction of Colles fracture and other distal forearm injuries. They are also useful in holding position allowing the surgeon freedom to apply long arm casts or posterior splints.

Application. Generally, the patient is placed supine with the elbow flexed at 90 degrees. The arm is commonly abducted, and the elbow protrudes over the edge of the table or stretcher. Two or preferably three fingers are placed in the trap device which should be suspended from a secure overhead position such as the pipe provided in the ceiling of most emergency rooms (Fig. 28). An intravenous pole can certainly be utilized, but care must be given to be sure that this is secured to the ground and not likely to tip.

Radial angulation is obtained by attaching the finger traps to the small and ring fingers (Fig. 28A). If a straight pull is required, the finger traps generally attach to the index and middle fingers (Fig. 28B). If slight ulnar angulation is desired, then the thumb and index finger are used (Fig. 28C). In this particular traction, the area of the forearm from the tip of the fingers to above the elbow is well exposed, and it is possible for a well molded cast to be applied by a single surgeon.

Risks. In spite of its many benefits there are two major risks in the use of finger traps. First, excessive time in the finger trap will lead to loss of skin on the side of the digit or necrosis of the finger tip. Our upper limit is 20 min. Second, excessive weight of over 5 lbs applied as countertraction can rapidly lead to loss of skin or even lacerations beneath the wire finger traps.

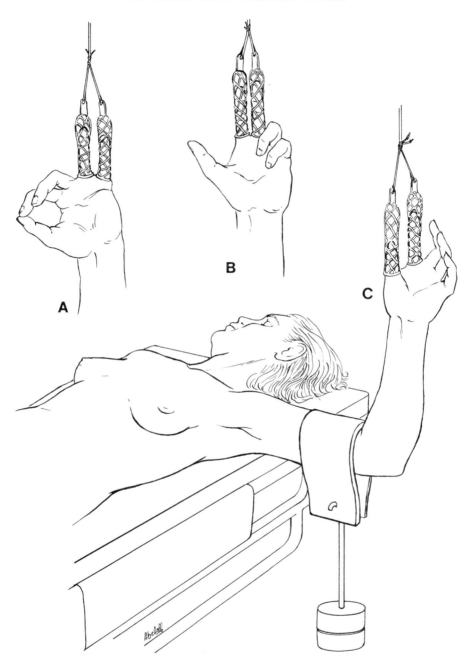

Fig. 28: Finger trap traction.
   28A: Finger trap applied to increase radial deviation of the head.
   28B: Finger trap positioned for a straight pull.
   28C: Finger trap applied to increase ulnar deviation.

REFERENCES

1. Blount, W.P.: Fractures in Children; William & Wilkins, Co., 1955
        Baltimore, Maryland

2. Dunlop, J.: Transcondylar Fractures of the Humerus in Children;
        J.B.J.S. No. 21:59, 1939.

3. Griffiths, D.L.: Volkmann's Ischemic Contracture; Brit. J. Surg.,
        28:239, 1940.

4. Hartman, T.J.: Fracture Management: A Practical Approach; Lea and
        Febiger, Philadelphia, 1978.

5. Ormandy, L.: Olecranon Screw for Skeletal Traction of the Humerus;
        Amer. J. of Surg., 127:615, 1979.

6. Tachdjian, M.O.: Pediatric Orthopaedics; W.B. Saunders Co.,
        Philadelphia, 1972.

7. Vichare, N.A.: Fractures of the Humeral Shaft Associated with
        Multiple Injuries; Injury, 5: 279.

CHAPTER 5

Traction for Pelvic or Acetabular Fractures

<u>Pelvic Sling Suspension</u>

<u>Indications</u>. Pelvic sling traction has been popularized for the treatment of minimally displaced pelvic fractures which require only mild compressive forces to maintain reduction. In fact, it seems to offer little advantage over bed rest with good nursing care. The major drawback in pelvic sling traction is the use of the bedpan. It becomes necessary to cut out the back of the sling and to frequently move the sling cephalad when attempting to get the patient on or off of the bedpan. Even with a Bradford frame, this represents a considerable difficulty and a moderate drawback to the use of this device.

<u>Application</u>. The patient is placed supine on the bed and a large piece of felt is cut so that its width reaches from the level of the ischial tuberosity to above the iliac crest. In length, it should be long enough to extend across the patient's back and well up either side, at least 6 or 8 inches above the patient. With great care, this is passed beneath the pelvis and brought up on either side of the patient. At this point, the felt is perforated along its margin and a metal spreader is inserted into the perforations. From each side, a traction line is run up and across the midline so that both lines form a large X directly above the patient's pelvis. Approximately 10 lbs of traction is initially placed on the pelvic sling as a whole, but this is frequently increased to 15 or 20 lbs, seldom exceeding 25 lbs (Fig.29A&B).

<u>Risks</u>. The major risk associated with this traction is that associated with any pelvic fracture. Shock, bladder or urethral compromise, and displacement of the fracture are all carefully watched for in these patients. For this reason, the manipulation required in getting the patient on and off of the bedpan is especially concerning and represents the major drawback of this traction system. Careful attention must be directed to the fit of the sling, and adequate allowance must be made for the patient to clear the sling for bowel movements and bathing.

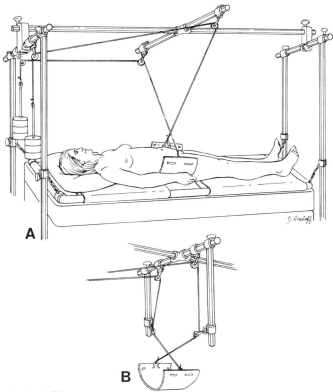

Fig. 29A: Pelvic Sling.
     29B: Minor modification to sling to increase lateral compressive
           forces. Pelvic sling traction with Bradford frame to facili-
           tate the use of bed pan.

* * * * * * * * * * *

Upper Femoral Skeletal Traction For Acetabular Fractures (Fig. 30)

     Indications. Several traction options are possible with fractures
of the acetabulum. An appropriate choice depends upon which portion of
the acetabulum is broken, as well as the direction and magnitude of displacement of fracture fragments. If primarily the cephalic portion is
broken, it is likely that the fracture force was directed cephalad.
The traction force should then be applied to pull the limb in the opposite direction. If no fragment displacement is present, light weight
skin traction such as Buck's (Fig. 31) or Russell's (Fig. 32) with the
lower limb in neutral abduction-adduction should suffice. If significant displacement has occurred or the degree of comminution indicates
instability, more forceful skeletal traction is indicated. This can be
achieved with traction applied to a pin inserted across the distal femur
(Fig. 37) or proximal tibia (Fig.38).

If the injury is a posterior fracture-dislocation, 90 degrees skeletal traction is more appropriate (Fig. 35).

If displacement of acetabular fragments has resulted from the femoral head being driven medially, centrally, or anteriorly, traction laterally on an eyelet screw in the proximal femur is preferred.

Application. The eyelet screw is inserted by an operative technique similar to that used in nailing a fracture of the femoral neck. With the patient lying supine, the trochanteric area and lateral aspect of the proximal thigh are surgically prepped. A small incision is made over the posterolateral thigh several finger breadths distal to the tip of the greater trochanter. The screw is aimed up the femoral neck. The location, alignment, and depth of insertion of the screw should be confirmed by x-ray control.

Due to the pain usually caused by moving a patient with a pelvic or acetabular fracture for bedpan placement or linen change, a fracture bed with Bradford frame is recommended. The patient may be transferred to the fracture bed after insertion of the screw.

Since the traction force is directly laterally and distally with the traction line routed from the screw to a pulley on an outrigger in a line approximately 45 degrees to the limb, precautions should be taken to prevent the patient from being pulled out of bed. When a fracture bed with Bradford frame is used, a bedside attached to the mattress frame cannot be used since the mattress frame moves vertically independently of the Bradford frame. This pole is a satisfactory substitute for a bedside and does not interfere with the traction line as the mattress is lowered.

Undesirable sliding of the patient to the traction side can also be inhibited by tilting the bed sideways. For this purpose, a small block may be placed under each wheel on the involved side. Five-pound cast iron traction weights are especially suitable for this purpose due to their size, shape, and availability. One weight should be inverted and placed on the floor beside each of the two caster wheels on the traction side of the bed. This side of the bed is then lifted and each weight slid under the adjacent caster wheel. The wheel is prevented from rolling off of the weight by the concavity on the bottom, which is now uppermost. The tilt of the bed achieved by this technique is adequate to maintain the patient in the proper position and is reasonably comfortable.

Relocation of the femoral head and the acetabulum may be attempted either by applying 20 to 25 lbs weight to the traction line or by manipulating the lower limb and subsequently applying 10 to 20 lbs to maintain reduction. Either technique is based on the hope that as the femoral head is repositoned, the acetabular fragments will follow it into their appropriate position under the influence of the stretched joint capsule and ligamentum teres and the relatively negative pressure created by extraction of the femoral head. If the acetabulum does not constitute itself, one may be able to replace and transfix the fragments surgically, particularly if they are few and large. If this is not feasible, replacement arthroplasty may be appropriate.

Risks. Extension of infection into the proximal femur, hip joint, and fractured pelvis from the soft tissues around a percutaneous trochanteric traction device can occur and is a serious complication. To avoid this problem, the condition of the skin about the screw should be carefully monitored. If evidence of infection develops, the traction device should be removed and appropriate treatment rendered.

In the author's experience, skeletal traction on the proximal femur by a Kirschner wire or Steinmann pin traversing the greater trochanter anteroposteriorly is more likely to result in an infection of this type than an eyelet screw used as described.

In order to reduce the occurrence of thrombophlebitis, sacral pressure sores, and other problems associated with prolonged recumbency, a degree of active motion by the patient should be encouraged. These movements may be assisted by providing the patient with a trapeze and instructing him in its use.

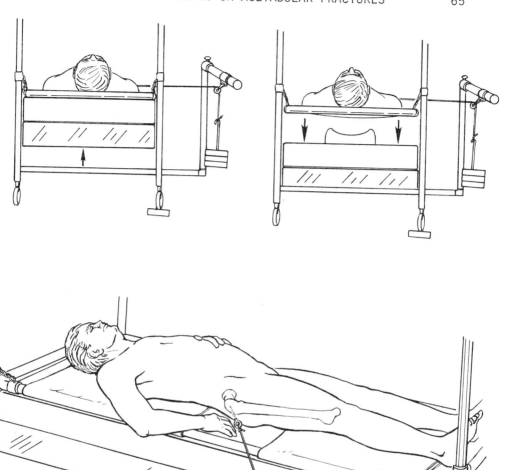

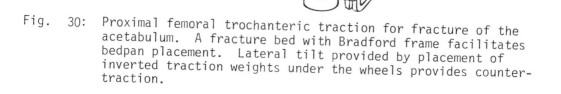

Fig. 30: Proximal femoral trochanteric traction for fracture of the acetabulum. A fracture bed with Bradford frame facilitates bedpan placement. Lateral tilt provided by placement of inverted traction weights under the wheels provides counter-traction.

REFERENCES

1. Compere, C.L.: Pictorial Handbook of Fractures Treatment; Chicago,
        The Year Book Publishers, Inc., 1958.

2. Courtial, D.C.: How to Care for the Patient with Pelvic Traction;
        Hospital Management, Aug: 16, 1971.

3. DeWitt, R.F.: A Method of Treatment Used in Fracture of the Ace-
        tabulum; J.B.J.S. No. 24, pp. 690, 1942.

4. Hamilton, F.G., Cahoy, H.E.: The Reduction of Central Fracture
        Dislocation of the Hip; Bull. Hurou Road Hospital 7:4, 1961.

5. Holm, C.L.: Treatment of Pelvic Fractures and Dislocations; Clin.
        Ortho. and Related Research. No. 97, 1973.

6. Schmeisser, G.: A Clinical Manuel of Orthopaedic Traction Techniques;
        W.B. Saunders Co., 1963.

7. Wilde, V.J.: Installation, Use and Evaluation of a Home Care Pelvic
        Traction Device; Amer. Corr. Ther. J., March - April:56, 1974.

CHAPTER 6

Lower Extremity Traction

Traction For Femoral Fractures (Fig. 31)

Indications. Buck's extension to the lower limb is widely used for conditions of the lower back, hip, femur, or knee for which partial immobilization with light traction force is desired. Examples are low back pain, nondisplaced acetabular fractures, following reduction of dislocation of the hip, following hip joint arthroplasty, before and after open reduction and internal fixation of fractures at any level of the femur, to protect an injured knee, and to resist or overcome mild hip or knee flexion contractures. Although Buck's extension rarely reduces a fracture or dislocation in an adult patient, properly used, it provides a measure of comfort. It also instantly alerts uninformed personnel that the patient has a significant skeletal problem and tells them which limb is involved.

Application. Satisfactory Buck's extension or other skin traction can be applied with ordinary adhesive tape, an elastic bandage, a length of cord, and a spreader consisting of any light rectangular object of suitable dimensions. Most surgeons prefer to use commercially available kits intended for a single application and containing all necessary components in appropriate sizes. Adhesive tape marketed for this specific purpose consists of synthetic sponge padding backed with soft strong fabric. The face of the padding is either coated with an adhesive gum or relies upon the friction of the sponge surface to secure purchase. All of these materials irritate skin; whenever possible, they should not be applied over an area where insertion of a skeletal traction pin or an incision might later be necessary. If Buck's extension is applied for temporary immobilization of a fractured hip, or shaft of the femur, the tape should not extend above the knee. If surgery is not anticipated, the tape may run higher, but should not extend as high as the level of the fracture. If it extends above the level of the fracture, part of the pull on the tape will be transmitted via the soft tissues to the proximal fragment rather than just the distal fragment, thereby reducing efficiency. The strips of tape should not overlap in front or in back of the extremity; instead, a small strip of skin should be left uncovered to permit swelling and to prevent constriction should the tape slip down the extremity. Within these limitations, the traction tape should cover as much skin as possible in order to minimize the pull on each square unit of skin surface.

Shaving the extremity prior to application of the tape is usually

67

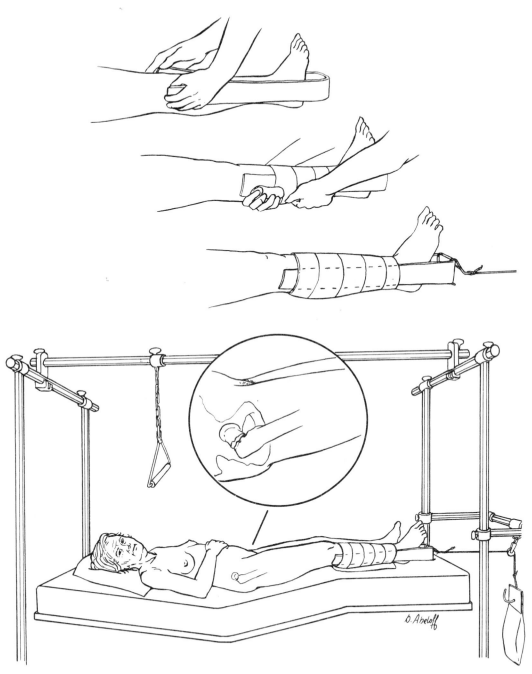

Fig. 31: Buck's extension is widely used for conditions of the lower back, hip, femur, or knee for which partial immobilization with light traction force is desired.

not necessary to secure good adhesion, provided the skin is well cleaned. On the other hand, if the limb is particularly hirsute, removal of
tape is likely to be particularly uncomfortable. For this reason, the
author prefers to shave such extremities, preferably with electric hair
clippers, with care to avoid scratches or very close shaving which are
likely to cause folliculitis under the tape. Tincture of benzoin, de-
spite its traditional use in many institutions, may not improve the bond
of most kinds of tape adhesive. Furthermore, it sometimes irritates
rather than protects the skin. Therefore, unless specified by the manufacturer of the specific type of tape, its use is not recommended. The
elastic bandage used to improve the bond of tape to skin must be wrapped
snugly enough to do the job, but without wrinkles and not so tightly as
to cause distal swelling. A few turns of the bandage about the foot inside the free ends of the traction tape also reduces this problem. The
malleoli and particularly the tendo Achilles usually need some protective padding.

     Several types of spreaders are available, each with minor advan-
tages (see Fig. 32). The traction tape should be divided into separate
medial or lateral strips only if a spreader with buckles is used. Selection of a spreader with width slightly wider than the ankle is more
important than design.

     Risks. Distal edema, vascular obstruction, peroneal nerve palsy,
and skin necrosis over bony prominences and over the Achilles tendon are
occasional complications of Buck's traction. When such problems are
suspected, the elastic bandages should be removed, the skin inspected,
and the limb rewrapped more loosely. Skin traction tape is likely to
slip or blister the skin if greater than 10 lbs are applied. Such low
force levels are not likely to reduce fractures in adults and may not be
adequate to maintain reduction achieved by manipulation. Attempts to
increase the efficiency of the traction tape by wrapping the elastic
bandages more tightly should be avoided.

Split Russell's Traction (Buck's With Sling) (Fig. 32)

     Indications. A sling may be added behind the knee, lower thigh, or
upper leg whenever greater knee or hip flexion or thigh support is desired than can be achieved with Buck's extension. This form of traction
is useful for the same conditions as Buck's extension; it may also be
used for reduction and immobilization of fractures of the middle and
distal thirds of the femur in children.

     Application. The skin traction is applied as described previously
for Buck's extension.

     The support sling must not be constrictive. Length and width must
be carefully selected both to avoid constriction and to distribute pressure as desired. If the material tends to bunch or pucker causing excessive local pressure, multiple spreaders should be used. Support

slings are commercially available; however, one can be fabricated easily from a ½-inch thick strip of saddlers felt approximately 6 inches wide and 18 inches long. It is slit near each end to receive one or more spreader bars.

The optimal position of pulleys, alignment of traction and suspension lines, and weight selection are most easily achieved by supporting the limb in a position which provides reasonable comfort for the patient and seems to align the fracture fragments and maintains a slight anterior bow of the femur. Ideally, the patella and foot are pointed toward the ceiling and the knee and hip are each flexed slightly. Weights are then added to the weight carriers until the limb is maintained in position without manual support. The thigh and leg supports of the mattress frame are then adjusted with a pillow under the thigh, knee, or leg to supply additional stability. Neither the force on the traction weight or the suspension sling should exceed 10 lbs. If the system is applied for a fracture of the shaft of the femur, the support sling must lie primarily underneath the distal fragment and its suspension line should be perpendicular to the longitudinal axis of the distal fragment.

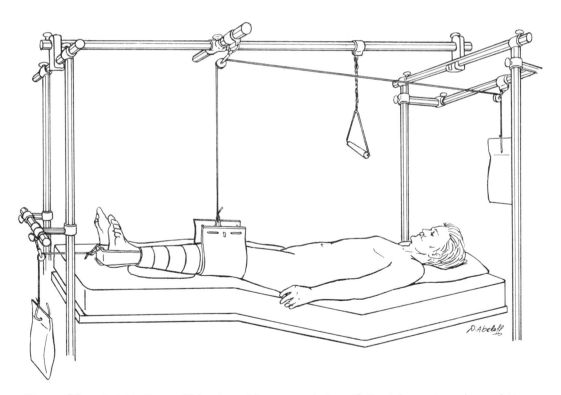

Fig. 32: Split Russell's traction consists of Buck's extension with a counterweighted support sling.

Risks. In addition to the risks of Buck's traction discussed previously, the thigh sling may displace and angulate the fracture. The
support sling is likely to cause valgus malalignment of a fracture of
the shaft of the femur if the patient lies with his limb in external
rotation.

Knee and Hip Exerciser (Fig. 33)

Addition of a cord and handle is a useful modification whenever
active assistance of knee and hip flexion and extension is desired.
This involves routing an additional piece of traction cord from the
support sling through one or two additional pulleys to a handle placed
within the patient's reach. A spreader bar or bundle of tongue depres-
sers taped together makes a satisfactory handle. The sling must be positioned to facilitate knee flexion. Bed adjustments for knee and leg
support must be lowered to facilitate knee extension. The traction line
and support sling line must both be cut long enough to permit the desired range of motion.

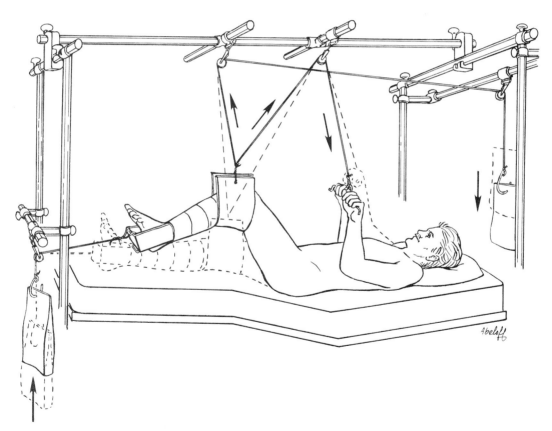

Fig. 33: Knee and hip exerciser.

Low Angle Bryant's Traction (Bilateral Uphill or High Angle Buck's)

A hybrid traction system which is very useful for treatment of a fractured shaft fracture in an infant or small child has evolved from combining features of Bryant's (gallows) traction and Buck's traction (Fig. 34). Bryant's traction involves vertical suspension of both lower limbs with the hips flexed 90 degrees and the knees extended. Although effective in immobilization and treatment of a fractured shaft of the femur in a small child, its use entails a definite risk of compromised circulation and resultant Volkmann's contracture of the foot and lower leg. This may involve either the injured or the opposite limb.

Buck's traction is unilateral and involves a horizontally aligned traction force with the involved hip and knee extended or only slightly flexed. Bilateral application improves immobilization but a small child slides toward the foot of the bed until the spreaders press against the pulleys. Effective traction on the fractured femur is then lost.

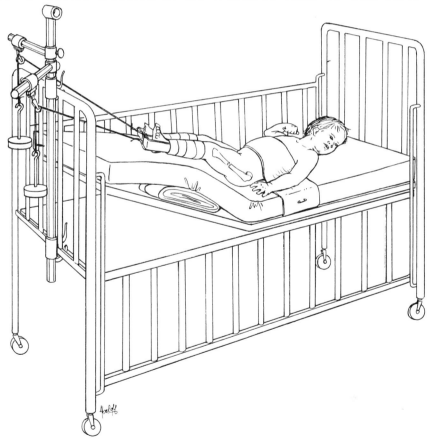

Fig. 34:   Low angle Bryant's, bilateral uphill or high angle Buck's traction.

A satisfactory compromise can be achieved by raising the lower half of the mattress high enough to supply effective countertraction, but low enough to minimize risk of compromised circulation. If the bed cannot be adjusted to create an appropriately curved support surface for the lower limbs, firm padding such as folded sheets placed between the mattress and the springs will serve the same purpose. Placed beneath the mattress it is more likely to remain in the proper position than if placed on top.

It is especially important that the feet of any child in any form of skin traction be checked frequently for pallor, loss of sensation, loss of toe motion, or other signs of circulatory embarrassment, particularly during the first 48 hrs. If such signs occur, the circumferential dressings must be loosened, the traction force reduced, and the leg lowered to a level at which circulation is restored.

Ninety-90 Degrees Traction Through Distal Femur (Fig. 35)

Indications. This form of traction is especially useful in the management of subtrochanteric fractures and fractures in the proximal third of the shaft of the femur. It is especially useful in children in the general age group of 5 to 15 years. Its usefulness extends to mid shaft fractures in children under 10 years old. Since this traction system can tolerate considerable patient abuse while maintaining fragment alignment, it is especially useful in uncooperative children.

It is less frequently indicated in young or middle-aged adults because in this age group it may result in some degree of prolonged hip flexion contracture or knee stiffness.

It is peculiarly useful in elderly, bedridden, or semi-bedridden adults, including ones with excessive anterior bowing of the femur, with or without Paget's disease. In this group, a minor irreversible hip and knee flexion contracture usually already exists and is not significantly aggravated by this type of traction. After a few days of adjustment, patients are remarkably comfortable for long periods of time. This arrangement is not conducive to pressure sores and, in fact, can be used to prevent them.

Finally, this system in unilateral or bilateral configurations is useful in treating severe burns or other problems involving skin loss over the buttocks and lower limbs.

Application. Flexion of a proximal fragment to a vertical or near vertical position is characteristic of subtrochanteric and proximal femoral shaft fractures. The position of this fragment is not easily controlled.

Alignment is most easily achieved by suspending the distal fragment vertically in alignment with the proximal one. This is achieved by sus-

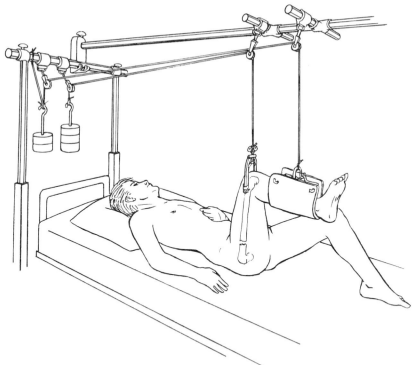

Fig. 35:   Ninety-90 degrees traction through distal femur.

* * * * * * * *

pending the limb by a skeletal pin across the distal femoral metaphysis
and by a sling under the calf, the limb being positioned with the knee
and hip flexed to 90 degrees.

     The traction wire or pin must be inserted with particular care in
view of the extent of the suprapatellar pouch anteriorly and proximally,
the neurovascular structures behind the distal femur, and, in children,
the presence of the distal femoral epiphyseal plate. In general, the
pin should pass along or slightly posterior to the midcoronal plane of
the femoral shaft (Fig. 36). It should also pass just proximal to the
adductor tubercle in order to avoid engagement of the collateral ligaments. When swelling has obscured the landmark, it is helpful to re-
member that it lies almost at the level of the proximal pole of the
proximal pole of the patella in the relaxed and extended knee. During
actual insertion of the wire, the knee should preferably be flexed in
order to draw the periarticular soft tissues into the position they will
occupy while the limb is in traction, thereby reducing pressure necrosis
of the skin around the wire.

     A Kirschner wire should be used only if it is of the largest size,
i.e. 0.62 inch thick, not threaded or nicked, and securely fastened to
a Kirschner wire tractor bow which is tightened forcefully. To prevent

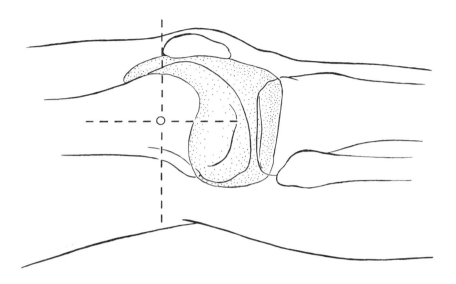

Fig. 36:   Preferred site for insertion of traction pin through distal
             femur.

* * * * * * * * *

unintentional disengagement of the wire from the tractor bow, the two
wire grippers or the ends of the bow arms should be firmly closed and
the ends of the wire bent to lie along the outside of the bow arms
thereby locking the grippers. In this position, the wires should be
taped to the bow so that their sharp tips are not exposed and the grippers cannot be inadvertently released.

      If a Steinmann pin is used in an adult, it should be at least 1/8
inch thick. Although a smaller sized pin may not break, bending becomes a problem. A Steinmann pin bow should be used with a Steinmann
pin rather than a Kirschner wire bow. The tips of the Steinmann pin
should be clipped close to the bow and capped. Kirschner wires are
usually provided with a diamond shaped tip which facilitates penetration of bone when used in a drill. Larger Steinmann pins may have a
trochar tip. Pins with this tip are more easily hammered than drilled
across the bone. In either case, counter force provided by an assistant
pressing against the limb from the opposite side is helpful.

      The support sling for the leg should be sufficiently long, thick,
and soft to support it without excessive local pressure. Although

satisfactory slings are commercially available, the appropriate size may be more easily obtained by cutting the sling out of a broad piece of ½-inch thick saddlers felt at the bedside. Spreaders may be oriented transversely, longitudinally, or both, in order to avoid excessive local pressure.

After attachment of the tractor bow and placement of the support sling, the traction framing including crossbars, pulleys, ropes, and weights should be assembled in anticipation of the limb being in the ninety-90 degrees position. The limb should then be lifted and supported manually in this position while the traction equipment is further adjusted and attached to maintain the limb in the appropriate position. The line from the tractor bow sustains most of the weight of the limb as well as any force required to overcome muscle spasm. The combined forces may be as little as 5 lbs in a small child or as much as 30 lbs in a large muscular adult. Ten to twenty pounds is the usual range. The support sling is counterbalanced with just enough weight to maintain the knee at 90 degrees.

If while suspended in traction the patient extends his knee, the calf support sling may displace toward his ankle. A check line consisting of an appropriate length of traction cord tied at one end to the support sling weight carrier and at the other end to the crossbar over the weight carrier, will prevent the support sling from rising higher than desired as the knee is extended. When the patient relaxes, his calf will come to rest on the support sling in the original position.

A reasonable estimate of the adequacy of alignment is possible by careful visual inspection of the length and contour of the thigh and alignment of the entire limb. Rotary alignment and, to some extent, abduction and adduction can be controlled by alteration of the position of the overhead pulleys with respect to the midsagittal plane of the patient.

As early evidence of partial union is revealed by loss of tenderness and by radiologic appearance of immature callus, gentle active hip and knee exercises may be initiated. As more union occurs, traction force should be reduced and the traction and suspension pulley moved slowly toward the foot of the bed, thus reducing the degree of hip and knee flexion. Light skin traction (Buck's) applied to the lower leg and pulling toward the foot of the bed is of help in slowly extending the limb. Tilting the bed slightly head down may be necessary during this stage. When the thigh has been brought approximately half way down and the callus is sufficiently mature, a cast or cast brace may be applied with the patient still in traction. If desired, a spica box or equivalent frame may be placed under the patient to facilitate application of the cast or cast brace. The traction pin can be incorporated in the cast temporarily if desired. There is less chance of angulating a partially united fracture by this technique than by first removing the traction completely before applying the cast.

Risks. Some degree of knee stiffness and hip flexion contracture are the most frequent problems with this form of traction. These problems are especially frequent with adult patients.

Malplacement of the skeletal traction pin resulting in contamination of the knee joint, injury to the distal femoral epiphyseal growth plate, or neu rovascular injury are potentially serious problems and require immediate correction.

As with any percutaneous skeletal traction device, infection can occur. To avoid this complication, the condition of the skin about the traction pin should be carefully monitored and, if evidence of infection develops, the traction pin should be removed and appropriate treatment rendered.

Excessive traction force may result in valgus angulation or distraction at the fracture site. Unilateral ninety-90 degrees traction is very likely to result in valgus angulation if the traction force is great enough to lift the buttock on the involved side off of the bed.

Distal Femoral Traction In Extension (Fig. 37)

Indications. This traction system involves application of skeletal traction to the distal femur with alignment of the traction force in the longitudinal axis of the lower limb with the hip and knee minimally flexed. If forces of 10 lbs or less are desired with the limb in the same position, Buck's extension is preferable. If forces between 10 and 15 lbs are desired and if knee joint pathology is absent, proximal tibial skeletal traction in extension is preferable. Distal femoral traction in extension is the best choice when strong traction is desired. Examples are fractures of the pelvis or acetabulum with cephalad displacement which might be pulled into place by strong longitudinal traction on the lower limb. As mentioned previously, lateral femoral traction on an eyelet screw in the greater trochanter is more appropriate for medial or central acetabular fracture dislocation. Distal femoral skeletal traction in extension is useful following resection of the femoral head or removal of an endoprosthesis. Finally, it is a useful alternative to tibial skeletal traction for a femoral shaft fracture when co-existing knee pathology, ligament injury, or fracture of the proximal tibial metaphysis precludes tibial skeletal traction.

Application. Significant details pertaining to insertion of a Kirschner wire or a Steinmann pin in the distal femur and attachment of the tractor bow have been described in the chapter on ninety-90 degrees traction.

Since high traction forces are used (15 to 25 lbs) and are applied approximately in the long axis of the trunk, adjustments for countertraction are necessary to prevent the patient from sliding to the foot of the bed and losing effective traction. The bed must either be tilted

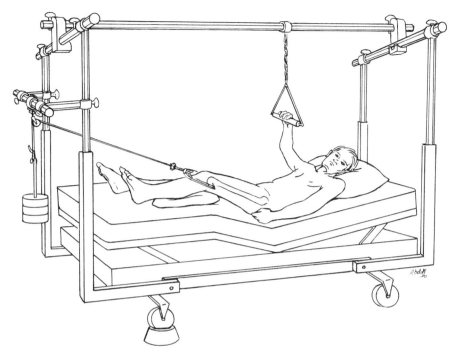

Fig. 37:   Distal femoral traction in extension.

* * * * * * *

or elevated on shock blocks to oppose the traction force. The knee
support of the mattress frame should be elevated slightly. A pillow
should be placed under the limb and positioned to prevent pressure on
the heel and to lift the knee enough to prevent contact between the
tractor bow and the skin on the front of the leg. The traction line
should be oriented in the long axis of the femur. The backrest should
be elevated slightly and the patient provided with a trapeze and taught
how to move about in bed and perform personal hygiene activities in a
manner campatible with his traction.

    If greater hip and knee flexion are desired, supporting the limb in
a balanced suspension system may be preferable to supporting it on a
pillow. These techniques are described in subsequent chapters with
tibial skeletal traction.

    Risks. Malposition of the traction pin and pin tract infection as
discussed previously with ninety-90 degrees traction are the major
risks with this form of traction.

    Knee joint stiffness is likely as a result of inflammation and scar-
ring of the soft tissues of the distal thigh from the percutaneous fem-

oral pin.

The skin over the tibial crest must be monitored for pressure by the traction bow. The skin over the lateral malleolus and heel should also be monitored closely to prevent or treat pressure sores.

Proximal Tibial Traction In Extension

Indications. Proximal tibial traction is most frequently used in the treatment of fractures of the distal two-thirds of the shaft of the femur in children over 10 years and in adults. In these circumstances, skin traction is usually unsatisfactory due to its limited force toler-ance. Distal femoral skeletal traction is unsatisfactory because the rotational moments about a femoral pin are unlikely to favor reduction of fractures in this portion of the femur.

Additional advantages of a proximal tibial traction pin site com-pared with a distal femoral pin site are the easier avoidance of the knee joint, the epiphyseal plate, and the soft tissues involved in knee joint motion.

Proximal tibial skeletal traction transmits traction forces across the knee joint. Therefore, it is contraindicated if the knee ligaments have been torn or relatively high force levels are used. For the latter reason it should not be used in a ninety-90 degrees position.

Application. Proximal tibial traction may be used in extension without any form of balanced suspension. Alternatively, it may be used with greater hip and knee flexion and in some form of balanced suspen-sion. Three modes of suspension are currently in common use. These various options will be individually discussed. Details of pin inser-tion are the same.

The ideal point for pin insertion of the wire or pin in an adult is approximately 1 inch posterior and 1 inch distal to the tibial tu-bercle (Fig. 38). With the patient supine and the lower limb prefer-ably supported on pillows, the proximal tibial area should be shaved and prepped as for any other surgical procedure. Following local in-filtration, the Kirschner wire or Steinmann pin should be driven trans-versely through the proximal tibial metaphysis, not the diaphysis. In a child, the proximal epiphyseal plate cephalad and the epiphyseal plate of the tibial tubercle anteriorly should be avoided. The branches of the peroneal nerve posteriorly are easily avoided. Occasionally, during insertion, the tip of the wire may creep anteriorly until the pin tra-verses the limb through the thick periosteum just in front of the tibial crest and routine x-rays may fail to reveal its incorrect location. The application of traction to a wire in this location will soon cause ex-cessive and persisting pain. Within a couple of days, the wire will lift away from the bone and stretch the skin. In these circumstances, the location of the wire should be promptly corrected. Incorrect wire

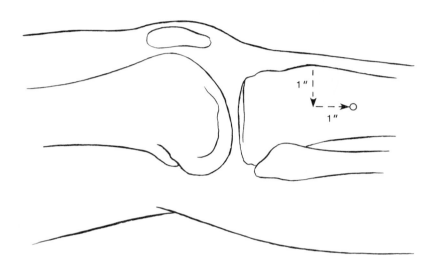

Fig. 38:   Preferred site for insertion of traction wire through
             proximal tibia.

                     * * * * * * *

placement can usually be prevented by inserting the wire well posterior
to the tibial crest and attempting to penetrate the bone with the wire
perpendicular to its surface.

    The largest size of Kirschner wire, i.e. 0.62 inch thick and with-
out threads or nicks, or a Steinmann pin approximately 1/8 inch thick
is usually satisfactory. Smaller Steinmann pins may not break, but
bending becomes a problem. Kirschner wires are usually provided with
a diamond-shaped tip which facilitates penetration of bone when used in
a drill. Larger Steinmann pins may have a trochar tip. Pins with a
trochar tip are more easily hammered than drilled across a bone. In
either case, counterforce provided by an assistant pressing against the
limb from the opposite side is helpful.

    A Kirschner wire tractor bow should always be used with a Kirsch-
ner wire and firmly tightened to stretch the wire in its long axis. To
prevent unintentional disengagement of the wire from the tractor bow,
the two wire grippers on the ends of the bow arms should be firmly
closed and the ends of the wire bent to lie along the outside of the
bow arms, thereby locking the grippers. In this position, the wires
should be taped to the bow arms so that their sharp tips are not exposed and the grippers cannot be inadvertently released. A Steinmann

pin bow and the protruding tips clipped close to the bow and capped.

The bed is adjusted and the traction equipment is arranged as for distal femoral traction in extension (Fig. 37). Adjustment for countertraction are necessary to prevent the patient from sliding to the foot of the bed and losing effective traction. The bed must either be tilted or elevated on shock blocks to oppose the traction force. The knee support of the mattress frames should be elevated slightly. A pillow should be placed under the limb and positioned to prevent pressure on the heel and lift the knee enough to prevent contact between the tractor bow and the skin on the front of the leg. When this system is used for a fracture of the femur, a traction force of 10 to 25 lbs is used and the traction cord is aligned approximately in the long axis of the proximal fragment of the femur.

If greater hip and knee flexion are desired, supporting the limb in a balanced suspension system may be preferable to supporting it on a pillow. Three appropriate balanced suspension systems are discussed later in this text. One of these involves a traction split and Pearson attachment. Another involves double slings. The third involves a cast brace.

Risks. Extension of infection into the proximal tibia from the soft tissues around the percutaneous traction wire or pin can occur. Rarely it may become a serious complication. To avoid this problem, the condition of the skin around the device should be carefully monitored. If evidence of infection develops, the wire or pin should be removed and appropriate treatment rendered. The development of troublesome infection is more likely if the wire or pin slips sideways. Sideways slip can be avoided by using a Steinmann pin with a short, threaded segment similar to the type used for the Hoffmann type external fixation apparatus. After insertion of the pin, the threaded segment should engage as much bone as possible and preferably not protrude through the skin. For this reason, fully threaded Steinmann pins are less satisfactory than partially threaded ones.

Contamination of the knee joint or injury to the epiphyseal plate or neurovascular structures is less likely when a proximal tibial wire or pin is used than a distal femoral one; however, anterior malposition of the wire or pin is more likely. This problem and its correction have been described earlier in this chapter.

Balanced Suspension With Traction Splint And Pearson Attachment

Indications (Fig. 39). Proximal tibial skeletal traction is especially useful in regaining or maintaining length following fractures of the distal two-thirds of the femur in older children and adults. If elevation of the limb above the surface of the mattress is required to correct angular malalignment, a counterweighted support system is appropriate. Traction splints with Pearson attachments have been widely used for this purpose and offer more precise control of fracture fragment

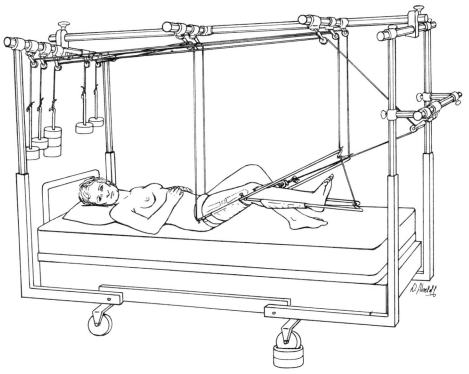

Fig. 39:   Proximal tibial skeletal traction with balanced suspension
            using a traction splint and Pearson attachment.

* * * * * * * *

alignment than suspension in double slings or plaster casts. This system is favored for cooperative adults with especially troublesome fractures with severe displacement, instability, or comminution.

    Disadvantages of this system include the more extensive amount of
equipment required and the complexity of the arrangement. The system
is especially vulnerable to maladjustment by uncooperative or confused
patients or unknowing personnel. Permissible patient movements are more
restricted and the system is less comfortable. Patients with bilateral
femoral shaft fractures or obesity are especially difficult to treat in
this system. Under these circumstances, suspension in double slings or
casts is preferable.

    Application. The proximal tibial skeletal traction pin is inserted
and the traction bow is attached as described previously (see Fig. S-13).

    All traction and suspension components should be collected and assem-
bled on the bed prior to moving the patient from his stretcher. The
traction splint selected should be of adequate length, breadth, and de-

sign. Ones with hinged half-rings may be reversed for use with either leg, and are superior for this purpose to the older, full-ring variety of the Thomas splint. If the half-ring is properly covered with neoprene or similar waterproof material by the manufacturer, additional padding is unnecessary and untidy. A Pearson attachment is clamped in the sides of the traction splint at a supracondylar level. The proximal portions of the splint and Pearson attachment are spanned with small hand towels pinned about each rod. These should be stretched tightly except near the half-ring, where considerable sag should be permitted to accommmodate the bulk of the proximal thigh. Commercial straps and pads are preferable to the towels if available. A felt or synthetic sheepskin pad placed on top of the towels will greatly enhance patient comfort. It should extend from proximal thigh to heel, be at least ½ inch thick and cut as wide as the splint.

The half-ring of the traction splint is then turned upwards, so that it will ultimately lie over the groin rather than posterior against the ischial tuberosity. The anterior position is preferred in balanced suspension because it facilitates use of the bedpan and does not promote undesirable flexion of the hip. Furthermore, countertraction is provided by tilting the bed rather than in impingement of the ring on the ischial tuberosity. Frequently, the half-ring tends to drop down spontaneously, thereby irritating the skin over the anterosuperior spine of the ileum. This tendency can be prevented by tying two pieces of traction cord from the sides of the half-ring to the screw clamps of the Pearson attachment (Fig. 40) or, if the thigh is thin, by tying a single cord from the center of the half-ring to the opposite end of the splint.

After the supporting splint has been dressed as described and placed on the bed, the overhead frame with appropriate crossbars and pulleys is assembled as illustrated in Figure 39. The crossbars intended to support the splint and leg should be placed directly above each end of the splint. In the case of a midshaft fracture, the crossbar for the main traction line should usually be clamped near the top of the 5½-foot upright poles. The main traction line and all four suspension lines are routed to the head end where the weights will clear the bed and hang freely when the foot of the bed is elevated on shock blocks and where the weights will not be disturbing passersby. Although the limb can be suspended by one suspension line attached at each end of the splint, a separate cord attached to each corner provides more precise control of rotation and is preferable if sufficient equipment is available. When attaching the two suspension cords to the proximal end of the splint, care must be taken to tie them in such a way they connot slip upward along the smooth side bars. DiCosola rope holders are helpful, or the cord may be tied about both side bars and half-ring (Fig. 41).

After application of dressings about the Kirschner wire and attachment of the tractor bow, the patient can be transferred from the stretcher to the bed. The injured extremity is lifted gently by pulling distally and upwards on the bow while supporting the lower leg. The trac-

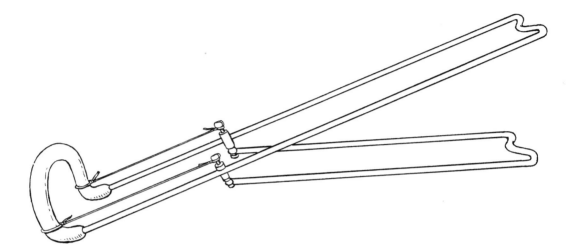

Fig. 40:   Anteflexion of the half-ring maintained by tying the sides
            of the half-ring to the screw clamps of the Pearson attach-
            ment.

                    * * * * * * * *

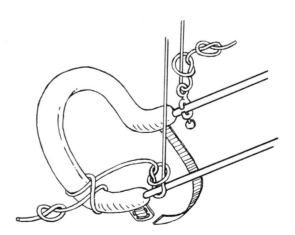

Fig. 41:   Alternate techniques for attachment of the two suspension
(continued on page 85)

Fig. 41: cords at the proximal end of the traction splint, to prevent
          distal slip of the cords along the side bars. DiCosola rope
          holder with slip knot at top; slip knot and clove hitch at
          bottom.

                    * * * * * * * *

tion splint with Pearson attachment, towels, pad, and supporting cords
is then slipped into place. After the main traction line is tied to the
tractor bow, a weight carrier is tied to the opposite end and 15 to 25
lbs of weights are placed on the carrier. Additional weights adequate
to lift the splint into a position which appears to align the fracture
fragments are attached to the carriers attached to the ends of the four
suspension cords. The distal ends of the traction splint and Pearson
attachment are connected by a short piece of cord. When the assembly is
properly adjusted and balanced, the half-ring does not press on the skin.

     If precautions are not taken soon after the patient is placed in
balance suspension, the splint may gradually slip distally on the leg.
This may be prevented by tying a piece of cord under slight tension from
the distal end of the splint to the Kirschner wire bow (Fig. 42).

     Both the traction and suspension systems are arranged somewhat
differently, depending upon the level of the fracture. In general, the
more proximal the fracture, the more the proximal fragment is flexed
anteriorly by the iliopsoas muscle. For this reason, when the fracture
is located in the upper third of the shaft, it is usually necessary to
orient the longitudinal axis of the distal fragment vertically in order
to align it with the sharply flexed proximal fragment. This orientation
is best obtained with ninety-90 degrees traction and with a distal femoral skeletal traction pin as shown in Figure 35.

     When the fracture lies in the middle third of femur, the
proximal fragment is longer and less flexion occurs; therefore, less
elevation of the distal fragment is required for reduction; 30 to 40
degrees is usually adequate. The main traction line should be aligned
with the longitudinal axis of the proximal fragment. This cord then
lies close to or in contact with the transverse part of the distal end
of the traction splint (Fig. 42A).

     When the fracture lies in the distal third or supracondylar area,
the distal fragment is short and is flexed posteriorly by the gastrocnemius muscle; therefore, the thigh need not be supported at a high angle,
but the knee should be flexed more sharply. The Pearson attachment
should be fastened to the side bars of the traction splint at the level
of the fracture, thereby creating a fulcrum around which the limb can be
pulled to help correct alignment. The main traction cord should be oriented horizontally or at a downward angle. (Fig. 42B).

     A device to support the foot in dorsiflexion is appropriate if any
weakness of ankle-foot dorsiflexion power is detected. Homemade dorsi-

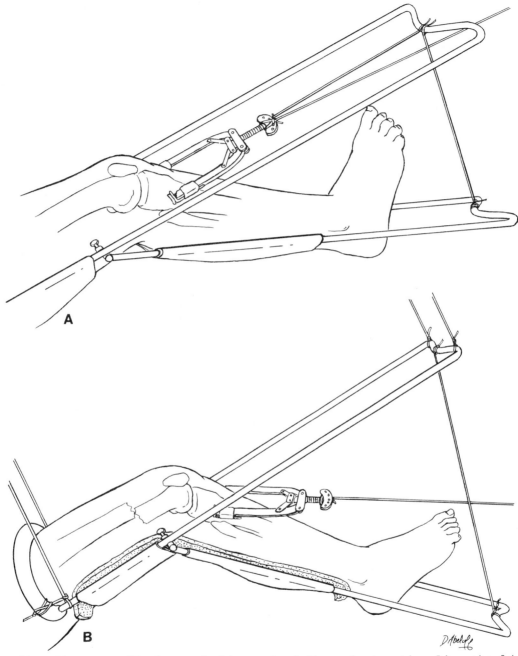

Fig. 42:   Knee flexion and alignment of the main traction line should
           be arranged according to the level of the fracture.
           (Figure legend is continued on page 87.)

Fig. 42A: In a midshaft fracture, the main traction line should be
             aligned upward and approximately in the longitudinal axis
             of the proximal thigh. A cord from the distal end of the
             splint to the tractor bow prevents distal displacement of
             the splint.
Fig. 42B: In a supracondylar fracture, the main traction line should
             be oriented horizontally or downward. Knee flexion should
             be increased.

* * * * * * * * * *

flexors can be as satisfactory as commercially available ones. One such
type is illustrated in Figure 43.   It consists of a plaster or isoprene stirrup which is supported against the ball of the foot by rubber
bands. It is fabricated by using a cardboard plaster box as an inside
mold. The width of the box should be at least 1 inch greater than the
breadth of the foot. A thick plaster or isoprene splint is draped over
the box. After the splint has set, it is padded with a 2-inch thick
foam and holes are made for rubber bands. The rubber bands should be
adjusted to support the ankle in a vertical position with light pressure
against the ball of the foot and to avoid pressure against the sides of
the foot; the stirrup must be rigid rather than flexible.

During convalescence, clinical and radiological examinations will
reveal the need for various adjustments. Alterations of the amount of
weight on the main traction line and other cords are usually necessary
at different stages of reduction. Occasionally, it is necessary to insert a small folded sheet or towel at the proper point under the thigh
to restore the normal anterior bow of the femur. If the fragments are
displaced medially or laterally, movement of the pulleys toward or away
from the midline is helpful in restoring alignment.

It should be appreciated that by pulling on a trapeze and pressing
downward on the mattress with the foot of his uninjured lower limb, the
patient may move himself vertically and longitudinally. Assistance of
his movements by an attendant should, of course, be performed by helping
to lift his trunk, not his leg. The balanced suspension system should
allow the limb to move easily with the patient. If the bed is not tilted adequately for countertraction, the patient must consciously maintain
a position toward the head of the bed. No attempt at turning from the
waist down is permissible.

As early evidence of some union is revealed by the loss of tenderness at the fracture site and by the radiological appearance of immature
callus, gentle knee and hip exercises may be initiated. These may be
assisted by an exercising cord tied to the distal end of the Pearson
attachment and routed through overhead pulleys to a handle within the
patient's reach (Fig. 44). A spreader bar or several tongue depres-
sors taped together makes a satisfactory handle.

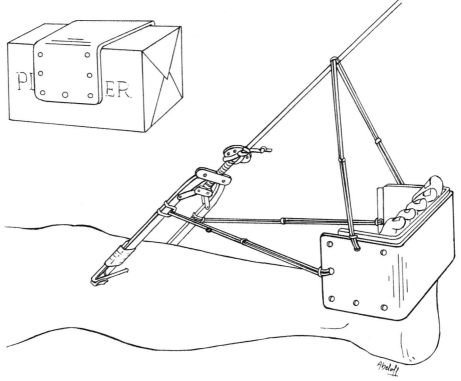

Fig. 43:   A homemade dynamic dorsiflexor can be made easily from a
            strip of isoprene or a plaster splint using a plaster box
            as a mold. Rubber bands linked together support the splint
            and resist plantar flexion.

                    * * * * * * * * * *

     When callus appears sufficiently mature, and there is no longer
motion at the fracture site, the traction splint and Pearson attachment
may be removed and a spica cast or cast brace applied with the patient
still in the tibial skeletal traction following which the traction may
be removed and the patient sent home to await more solid union.

     Risks. One of the more frequent complications of balance suspen-
sion in a traction splint with Pearson attachment is a foot drop in
association with pressure on the peroneal nerve behind the fibular head.
This is usually associated with distal displacement of the splint or
Pearson attachment.

     The traction pin site should be monitored for the same problems
mentioned previously in association with proximal tibial traction in
extension.

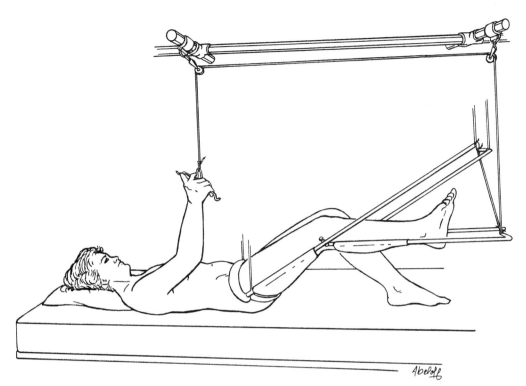

Fig. 44:   A cord tied to the distal end of the Pearson attachment and
routed through overhead pulleys to a handle helps the patient perform knee extension exercises.

* * * * * * * * * *

Balanced Suspension With Double Slings (Fig. 45)

Indications. Balanced suspension in double slings is a useful alternative to balance suspension in a traction splint and Pearson attachment for treatment of fractures of the distal two-thirds of the shaft of
the femur in older children and adults. It requires less equipment, is
easier to assemble, is more comfortable, and is adequate for treatment
of all but the most troublesome fractures, i.e. those characterized by
severe displacement, instability, or comminution. It is preferred for
patients with bilateral femoral shaft fractures or obesity. It allows
easy access to any part of the limb for treatment of concurrent wounds
or other skin problems. It facilitates application of a cast or cast
brace. Also, it is an easy method of stabilizing a fracture and maintaining limb length pending open reduction and internal fixation.

Application. The proximal tibial skeletal traction pin is inserted and the tractor bow attached as described previously (see Fig. 38).
The traction line pulleys, crossbars and weights are arranged and the

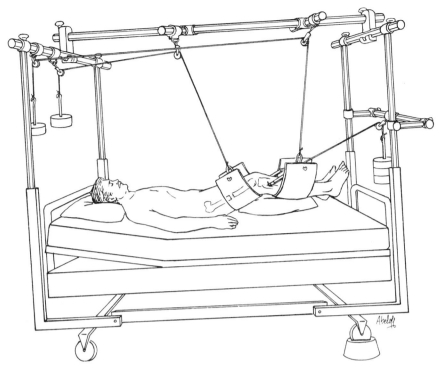

Fig. 45:   Proximal tibial skeletal traction with balanced suspension
             in double slings.

                  * * * * * * * * * * * *

bed tilted and adjusted as described for proximal tibial skeletal traction in extension.

     A thigh sling and a leg sling are used to suspend the limb as illus-
trated in Figure 45.   Commercially available suspension slings may be
used or they may be fabricated at the bedside from a sheet of ½-inch
thick saddlers felt. The thigh sling should be wide enough to support
the distal femoral shaft fragment. It should not extend so far proximal
that it increases flexion of the proximal fragment. The leg sling
should be wide enough to support the entire leg. The thigh sling must
be long enough to pass around the thigh and accept one or more spreaders.
The leg sling must be long enough to reach around the leg and the tractor bow and still accept one or more spreaders. If the slings appear
constrictive, multiple spreaders should be used to distribute pressure
evenly (see Fig. 35). The crossbar and pulley for suspension of the
thigh sling should be placed approximately over the hip joint. The
crossbar and pulley for the leg sling should be placed approximately
over the ankle. Weights should be added to the weight carriers on these
lines until the limb is lightly supported over the mattress. Fine ad-

justment of the weights,sling, and pulleys are then made until the limb appears properly aligned, at normal length and with a slight anterior bow of the thigh. The patella and foot should be pointed toward the ceiling and the hip and knee each flexed 20 to 30 degrees.

The traction and suspension systems are arranged somewhat different-ly depending upon the level of the fracture. In general, the more prox-imal fragment is flexed anteriorly by the iliopsoasis muscle. For this reason, when the fracture is located in the upper third of the shaft, it is usually necessary to orient the longitudinal axis of the distal fragment vertically in order to align it with the sharply flexed prox-imal fragment. This orientation is best obtained with ninety-90 degrees traction and the traction pin in the distal femur as shown in Figure 35. In general, the more distal the fracture, the less the proximal fragment is flexed anteriorly and the more the distal fragment is flex-ed posteriorly by the gastrocnemius muscle. When the fracture is locat-ed in the lower third or supracondylar area, angular displacement is aggravated by extension of the knee which may occur if the skeletal trac-tion pin is inserted too far distally or too much support is placed be-neath the leg (Fig. 46). Proximal placement of the traction pin with flexion of the knee and adequate support at the fracture lies in the middle third of the femur; the inclination of the main traction line should be elevated to coincide with the longitudinal axis of the proxi-mal fragment of the femur (see Fig. 42A). Hip flexion should be in-creased and knee flexion decreased.

A spring or elastic activated foot plate may be attached to the traction system to protect the power of the foot dorsiflexors as des-cribed previously (see Fig. 43).

It should be appreciated that by pulling on a trapeze and pressing downward on the mattress with the foot of the uninjured lower limb, the patient may move himself vertically and longitudinally. Assistance of his movements by an attendant should, of course, be performed by help-ing to lift his trunk, not his leg. The balanced suspension system should allow the limb to move easily with the patient. If the bed is not tilted adequately for countertraction, the patient must consciously maintain a position toward the head of the bed. No attempt at turning from the waist down is permissible.

During convalescence, clinical and radiological examinations will reveal the need for various adjustments. Alterations of the amount of weight on the main traction line and suspension cords are usually neces-sary at different stages of reduction. As early evidence of some union is revealed by the loss of tenderness at the fracture site and by the radiological appearance of immature callus, gentle knee and hip exercis-es may be initiated. When callus appears sufficiently mature and there is no longer motion at the fracture site, a spica cast or cast brace may be applied with the limb still in traction. The supporting slings may either be removed or incorporated in the cast. The skeletal trac-

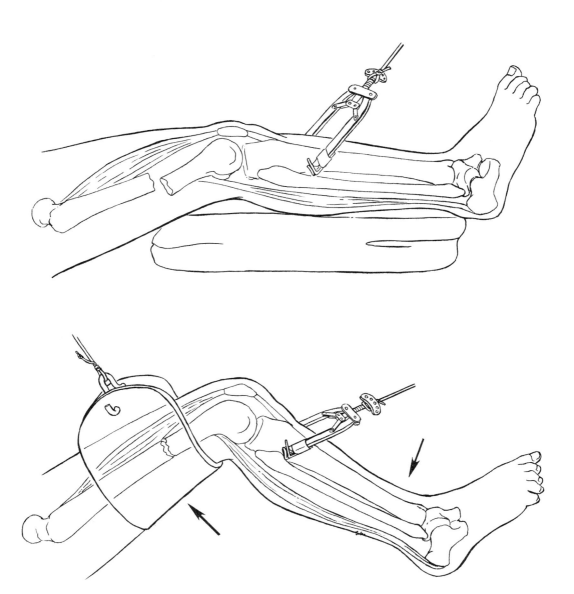

Fig. 46 : When the fracture is located in the lower third of the
            femur, angular displacement is aggravated by extension
            of the knee. More proximal placement of the traction
            pin with flexion of the knee and support at the fracture
            site facilitates reduction.

tion pin may also be removed immediately following application of the cast or left in situ for later removal.

Risks. Balance suspension in double slings is vulnerable to displacement of the slings by an uncooperative or confused patient. The skin around the traction wire must be carefully monitored for infection as discussed previously in association with proximal tibial traction in extension. The skin around the fibular head and over the Achilles tendon must also be monitored for excessive pressure from the support sling.

Balanced Suspension In Long Leg Cast Or Cast Brace (Neufeld)

Indications. Balance suspension in a cast or cast brace used in combination with proximal tibial traction is most useful for treatment of fractures of the distal two-thirds of the shaft of the femur in older children and adults (Fig. 47).   Compared with balanced suspension in a traction splint and Pearson attachment, this form of suspension offers the same advantages and disadvantages as double sling suspension. It has certain additional advantages. It is tolerant of extraordinary patient mobility and modification by personnel. Although an uncooperative patient may wriggle out of a traction splint and Pearson attachment or suspension slings, he cannot wriggle out of a plaster cast with a transverse percutaneous skeletal pin. Although the traction-suspension lines can be readily adjusted or detached, they can just as readily be readjusted or reattached. This system is especially useful with patients turned for pulmonary care or other reasons.

This system does not permit as good access to the skin over the lower limb as double sling suspension or as precise control of fragment alignment as the traditional type of balanced suspension in a traction splint and Pearson attachment illustrated in Figure 39.

Application. The system presented here for balanced suspension in a cast or cast brace is a modification of a system developed by Neufeld. Significant features of the Neufeld system include a pulley designed to roll along the traction pole mounted longitudinally over the patient's bed, suspension of the limb from this pulley, attachment of the main traction line to this pulley, encasement of the leg and skeletal traction pin in a plaster cast, unrestrained knee motion, and simplified detachment and adjustability of suspension line attachments to the cast.

The proximal tibial skeletal traction pin is inserted as described previously (see Fig. 38). With this system, a Steinmann pin is preferable to a Kirschner wire. Application of the plaster cast is facilitated by placing the patient in proximal tibial traction in extension with the bed and traction frame adjusted as in Figure 37. The knee rest is then lowered and the pillow is removed leaving the limb partially suspended by the traction system. A snug long leg cast is applied with slight flexion at the knee, a high proximal trim line, and careful molding of the proximal thigh segment. The main effort is to achieve optimal grasp of the thigh around the proximal fragment of the femur. The plaster should also grasp the Steinmann pin. Plaster is then removed from the cast at the knee joint medially, laterally, and posteriorly. A plaster connection is retained anteriorly between the thigh and leg sections for temporary stability. Polycentric cast brace hinges are then attached to the cast on the medial and lateral sides of the knee. Attachment points for the suspension lines are attached to the cast at the same time. Although special fittings are commercially available for this purpose, coathanger wire is satisfactory. If internal and external rotational capability is desired, these attachment wires should be mounted along the medial and lateral sides of the cast; otherwise, they can be mounted anteriorly along the midline of the thigh and leg. The lower ends of the suspension lines from the overhead rolling pulley should be tied to small S-hooks or snaps. These enable easy balancing adjustments. A new traction line is run from the rolling overhead pulley to a weight carrier at the end of the bed. Weights are shifted from the weight carrier on the old traction line to the new one until satisfactory balance and traction are achieved. The old traction line and Steinmann pin are clipped and capped. To enable knee motion, an elastic strap, section of surgical tubing, or a double-thickness heavy rubber Penrose drain, should be inserted in the line suspending the leg segment. Alternatively, knee motion may be enabled by attaching the two suspension lines to opposite ends of a long spreader, the center of which is suspended from the overhead pulley. After satisfactory suspension is achieved, the channel of plaster between the thigh and leg segments of the cast is divided transversely. The S-hooks on the lower ends of the suspension lines may then be shifted proximally or distally on the cast to promote either flexion or extension of the knee.

Finally, as union occurs, a knee flexion assist line similar to that shown in Figure 33 or a knee extension assist line analogous to that shown in Figure 44 may be attached if desired.

Risks. Malposition of the traction pin and pin tract infection as discussed previously in association with proximal tibial traction in extension may occur. Inspection of the pin site is impossible without cutting away plaster and padding; therefore, there is a tendency to delay confirmation of diagnosis and initiation of treatment. Fortunately, infection due to side slip of the pin is less likely in a cast.

Cast braces are frequently associated with swelling of the soft tissues about the knee. Rarely, it may be necessary to cut a channel down the thigh section of the cast and spread it slightly to facilitate venous return. Prefabricated commercially available quadrilateral cast brims of vinyl or plastic laminate may be used instead of plaster of Paris but are more likely to cause skin maceration.

Distal Tibial Skeletal Traction (Fig. 48)

Indications. Distal tibial skeletal traction has been found ex-

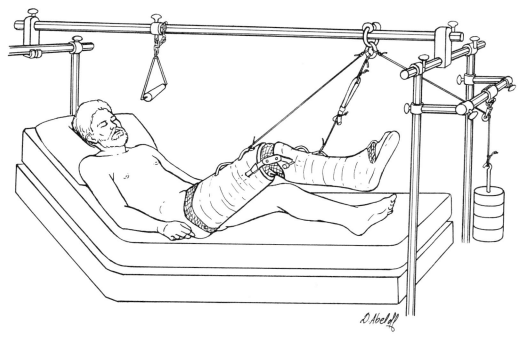

Fig. 47:   Proximal tibial skeletal traction with balanced suspension
             using a cast brace (Neufeld).

                    * * * * * * * * * *

tremely useful in the treatment of certain tibial plateau fractures.
When fragments are few and large, open reduction and internal fixation
with early motion may be the ideal treatment. If fixation is thought
not to be absolutely secure following such a procedure, the operation
may then be followed by either light traction or a plaster cast. If, on
the other hand, the fragments are too small and numerous to permit adequate repositioning by surgery, the initial use of traction offers certain advantages to casting. It is important that the traction system be
designed to enable early controlled active motion while traction forces
are maintained.

       Distal tibial traction is also useful in overcoming knee fexion
contractures and, to some extent, hip flexion contractures. Finally,
distal tibial skeletal traction is occasionally useful for tibial shaft
fractures temporarily to recover or maintain length for a short period
prior to definitive treatment by another technique.

       Application. Before inserting the skeletal traction pin, one should
check to see if the tractor bow is of adequate size to avoid pressure on
the sole of the foot when attached to the pin. The arms of Bohler-
Steinmann pin bows may usually be bent is such a way as to increase their
effective length. Since this is not true of Kirschner wire tractors,

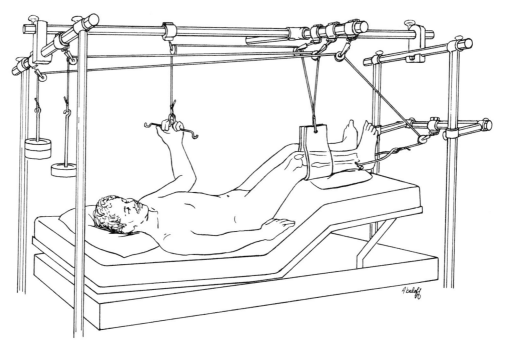

Fig. 48:   Distal tibial skeletal traction

* * * * * * * * * *

and since, with an adult male patient, the larger Kirschner wire tractors may not be long enough, one may prefer to use a Steinmann pin rather
than a Kirschner wire.

    In order to be certain of avoiding the tibiotalar joint, the pin
should be inserted 1¼ inches proximal to the tip of the medial malleolus
(Fig.   49). Care should be taken to miss the saphenous vein. Most
surgeons insert the traction pin with the intention of traversing only
the tibia. The author prefers to pass the pin through the center of the
lateral surface of the fibula, thereby avoiding injury to the peroneal
tendon sheaths, and continuing through the center of the medial surface
of the tibia, thereby avoiding the extensor tendons anteriorly as well
as the neurovascular bundle entering the tarsal tunnel posteriorly.

    When distal tibial skeletal traction is used for tibial plateau
fractures, the knee and leg adjustments of the mattress frame are elevated to maintain the limb in partial hip and knee flexion. Fifteen to
twenty pounds are applied to the main traction line in order to minimize
impaction forces across the knee joint. A felt sling, long enough to
encircle the knee and at least 6 inches wide is cut from ½-inch thick
saddlers felt and positioned around the proximal tibia and knee. This
sling is attached by separate lines to a 5-lb weight and to a spreader

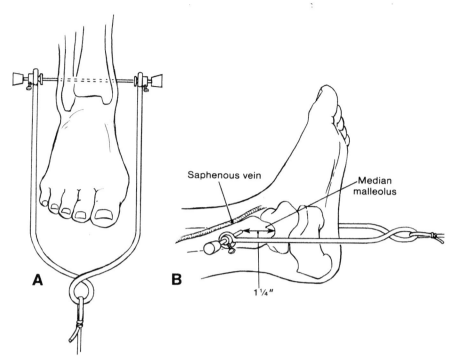

Fig. 49:   Preferred site for insertion of traction pin through the
            distal tibia and fibula.

                    * * * * * * * * *

within the patient's reach.

     With the patient adequately sedated and traction applied across the
knee, the surgeon can attempt to mold the plateau by interlacing his
fingers behind the knee and forceably compressing the sides of the proximal tibia with the heels of his hands. Within a few days after injury,
knee flexion and extension exercises should be encouraged. The patient
can assist himself in performing these exercises with the exerciser cord.
As knee flexion is regained, the knee rest may be lowered in stages to
regain extension.

     When distal tibial traction is used to stretch a knee flexion con-
tracture, a sling is not needed and the knee rest may be progressively
lowered.

     When distal tibial traction is used for maintenance of length and
temporary immobilization of a fracture of the shaft of the tibia, no
sling is required. The knee and leg rests should be elevated slightly
to maintain some hip and knee flexion with the leg aligned parallel with
the floor.

Risks. As with any percutaneous skeletal pin, the skin around the pin should be carefully monitored for evidence of infection. The skin around the proximal fibula and beneath the Achilles tendon and lateral malleolus should be carefully monitored for excessive pressure. Circulation in the leg and foot should be monitored for vascular compression. Tibial compartment pressure syndromes are not uncommon with these injuries and prompt surgical decompression may be necessary to salvage a useful limb. In such circumstances, the encircling sling should, of course, be removed and the traction force reduced.

Calcaneal Traction (Fig. 50)

Indications. Although treatment of a fracture of the calcaneus by traction is uncommon, and presents the disadvantage of contamination of the fracture hematoma by a percutaneous pin, this form of treatment is occasionally useful with a marked loss of the tuber joint (Bohler's) angle.

Occasionally, this form of traction is also useful temporarily for tibial shaft fractures to recover or maintain length prior to definitive treatment by some other technique.

Application. The correct spot for insertion of the pin may be measured from the malleoli, these being landmarks which can usually be palpated even in swollen feet (Fig. 51). Ideally, the pin should be inserted as far posterior as possible while still engaging sound bone. The tendons and neurovascular bundle passing behind the malleoli and, of course, the talocalcaneal joint are to be avoided. The traction pin should never be placed through the soft tissue space between the talus, calcaneus, and tendo-Achilles; this technique may lead to disasterous slough and infection.

The lower limb should be elevated slightly with slight flexion in the knee and a pillow beneath the leg avoiding pressure on the heel or tendo-Achilles.

Risks. Pain and swelling are frequent problems with calcaneal fractures. Constrictive dressing must be released and any localized pressure relieved in order to avoid skin slough.

Contamination and secondary infection of the calcaneal fracture hematoma from a percutaneous skeletal pin is a major risk in treating these fractures with this technique.

Transmetatarsal Suspension (Fig. 52)

Indications. Forefoot transfixation of the metatarsals with a skeletal traction pin, usually in association with a proximal tibial skeletal traction pin, is very useful for suspension of legs with severe burns and other soft tissue injuries. This technique greatly facilitates wound care. It may also be used to resist plantar flexion contractures.

Application. Insertion of the proximal tibial skeletal traction pin is described earlier in this text (see Fig. 38).

Following appropriate surgical prepping of the foot, a Kirschner wire or small gauge Steinmann pin is driven transversely across the foot distal to the tarso metatarsal joint of Lisfranc. Proper orientation is most easily achieved by inserting the pin or wire in the medial aspect of the base of the first metatarsal while aiming at the center of the fifth metatarsal shaft.

A tractor bow is attached to each of the skeletal pins. Suspension lines from the tractor bows may be routed vertically to pulleys on separate crossbars, one over the ankle and the other over the knee. In order to enhance foot dorsiflexion, the crossbars are brought closer together or both pulleys are placed on the same crossbar. Sufficient weight is placed on the weight carriers of each of these suspension lines to support the limb in the position desired.

Risks. Although pin traction infection is a serious potential complication in this system, the disabling nature of the conditions for which it is indicated justifies the risk.

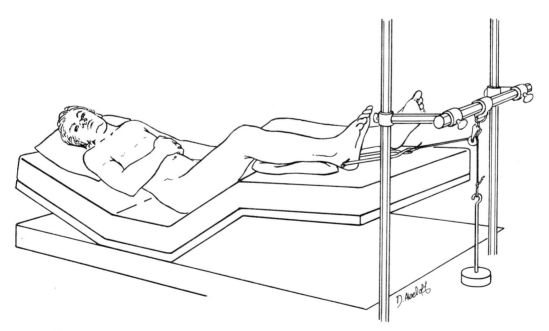

Fig. 50:   Calcaneal traction.

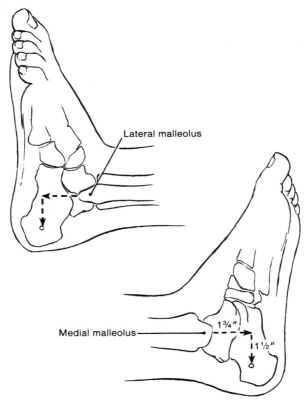

Fig. 51:   Preferred site for insertion of traction pin through the
            calcaneus.

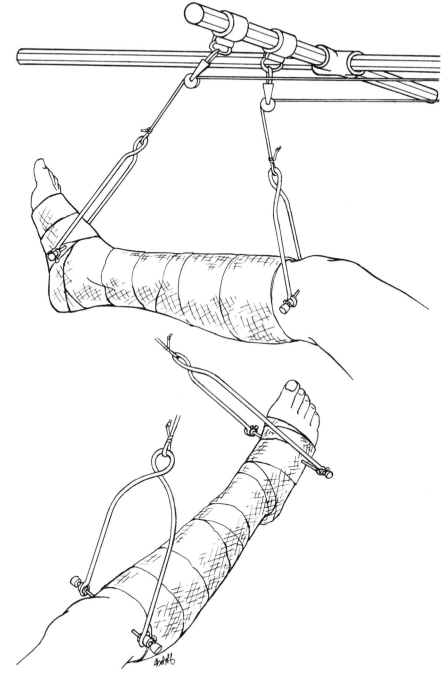

Fig. 52: Transmetatarsal and transtibial suspension for burn treatment and prevention of plantar flexion contracture.

REFERENCES

1. Apley, A.G.: Fractures of the Lateral Tibial Condyle Treated by
      Skeletal Traction and Early Mobilization: A Review of
      Sixty Cases with Special Reference to the Long-term Re-
      sults; J.B.J.S., 38B:699, 1956.

2. Anderson, R: Conservative Treatment of Fractures of the Femur;
      J.B.J.S., Vol. 49A, No.7, pp. 1371-1375, Oct. 1967.

3. Bohler, L.: Diagnosis, Pathology and Treatment; J.B.J.S., Vol.50A,
      No.8, pp. 1603-1617, Dec. 1968.

4. Brav, E.A.: The Use of Intramedullary Nailing for Non-union of the
      Femur; Clin. Orth. and Related Research, No.60, pp: 69-75,
      Sept.-Oct., 1968.

5. Brav, E. and Jeffress, V.: Fractures of the Femoral Shaft: A Cli-
      nical Comparison of Treatment by Traction Suspension and
      Intramedullary Nailing; Am. J. Surg., Vol.84, pp. 16-25,
      1952.

6. Buck, G.: An Improved Method of Treating Fractures of the Thigh;
      Trans. N.Y., Acad. Med. 2:233, pp. 1857-1863/Reprinted in
      Clin. Orth. and Related Research, No.140, pp. 2 - 11,
      May, 1979.

7. Cole, W.H.: Resutls of Treatment of Fractured Femurs in Children
      with Special Reference to Bryant's Overhead Traction;
      Arch. Surg., 5:702, 1922.

8. Conwell, H.E.: Acute Fractures of the Shaft of the Femur in
      Children; J.B.J.S., 11:593, 1929.

9. Dameron, T., and Thompson, H.: Femoral Shaft Fractures in Children;
      J.B.J.S., 41A, No.7, pp. 1201-1212, Oct. 1959.

10. Ilfelo, R.W.: A Modified Half-Ring Splint and Combined Foot Sup-
      port and Exerciser; J.B.J.S., Vol.43A, No.1, pp. 139-140,
      Jan. 1961.

11. Kauffer, H.: Nonoperative Ambulatory Treatment for Fracture of the
      Shaft of the Femur; Clin. Orth., No.87, pp. 192-199,
      Sept. 1972.

12. Lee, W.E., and Veal, J.R.: The Russell Extension Method in the
      Treatment of Fractures of the Femur: A Review of the
      Anatomical Results Obtained in a Group of Fifty One Cases;
      Surg. Gyn. and Obst., 56:492, 1933.

13. Lewis, R.G.: Handbook of Traction, Casting and Splinting Tech-
        niques; J.B. Lipponcott Co., Philadelphia, 1977.

14. Lowery, T.M.: The Physics of Russell Traction; J.B.J.S., 17:174,
        1935.

15. Mays, J., and Neufelo, A.J.: Skeletal Traction Methods; Clin. Orth.
        and Related Research., No.102, pp. 144-151, July-Aug., 1974.

16. Mitcheltree, R.G., Messner, D.G., Odom, J.A., Brown, C.W.: A Ba-
        lancing Femoral Traction Suspension System; Clin. Orth.
        and Related Research. No.103, pp. 27-28, Sept. 1974.

17. Mooney, V., Nickel, V., Harvey, J.P., and Snelson, R.: Cast-Brace
        Treatment for Fractures of the Distal Part of the Femur;
        J.B.J.S., Vol. 52A:8, pp. 1563-1578, Dec. 1970.

18. Nicholson, J.T., Foster, R.M., and Heath, R.D.: Bryant's Traction:
        A Provocative Case of Circulatory Complications; J.A.M.A.,
        157:415, 1955.

19. Peltier, L.F.: A Brief History of Traction; J.B.J.S., Vol.50A,
        No.8, pp. 1603-1617, Dec. 1968.

20. Rascher, J., Nahigian, S., Malys, J., and Brown, J.; Closed Nailing
        of Femoral Shaft Fractures; J.B.J.S., Vol.54A, No.3,
        pp. 534-544, April 1972.

21. Rokkanen, P., Slates, P., and Vankka, E.: Closed or Open Intra-
        medullar Nailing of Femoral Shaft Fractures: A Comparison
        of Conservatively Treated Cases; J.B.J.S., Vol.51, No.2,
        pp. 313-323, May 1969.

22. Rowie, C.: The Management of Fractures in Elderly Patients is
        Different; J.B.J.S., 47A, pp. 1043-1059, July 1965.

23. Russell, R.H.: Fracture of the Femur: A Clinical Study; Brit. J.
        Surg. 11:491, 1924.

24. Sarmiento, A.: Functional Bracing of Tibial and Femoral Shaft
        Fractures; Clin. Orth., No.82, pp. 2-13, Jan.-Feb. 1972.

25. Schmeisser, G.: A Clinical Manuel of Orthopaedic Traction Tech-
        niques 1963; W.B. Saunders Co., Philadelphia, 1963.

26. Schofield, R.O.: Fracture of the Os Calcis; J.B.J.S., 18:566, 1936.

27. Sifmon, L.: Refracture of the Shaft of the Femur; J.B.J.S., Vol.
        46B, No.1. pp. 32-39, Feb. 1964.

28. Steinmann, F.: Zur Geschichte der Nagelextension; Zeitschr. Orth.
    Chir., 29:96, 1911.

29. Stewart, M., Sisk, D., and Wallace, S.: Fractures of the Distal
    Third of the Femur; J.B.J.S., Vol.48, No.4, pp. 784-807,
    1966.

30. Stryker, W.S., Fussell, M.E., and West, H.D.: Comparison of the
    Comparison of the Results of Operative and Non Operative
    Treatment of Diophyseal Fractures of the Femur at the
    Naval Hospital, San Diego, Over a Five Year Period. In
    Proceedings of the American Academy of Orthopaedic Sur-
    geons; J.B.J.S., Vol.52A, No.4, p. 815, June 1970.

31. Urist, M.R., and Quigley, T.B.: Use of Skeletal Traction for Mass
    Treatment of Compound Fractures: A Summary of Experiences
    with 4,290 Cases During World War II.; Drch. Surg.
    63: 834, 1951.

32. Wendel, A.: Extracapsular Fractures of the Femur in the Aged:
    A Contribution to the Merits of Russell Treatment;
    J.B.J.S., 13:616, 1931.

33. Winant, E.M.: The Use of Skeletal Traction in the Treatment of
    Fractures of the Femur; J.B.J.S., 31A:87, 1949.

A

Acetabular fractures (see also
         Pelvic or acetabular
         fractures), 61-66
   Buck's extension, 67

B

Back pain, low
   Buck's extension, 67
   Cotrel traction, 30
   inpatient pelvic belt traction,
         for conservative treat-
         ment, 38-39
Balanced suspension
   DiCosola rope holders, 83
   dynamic dorsiflexor, 88
   in a long leg cast or cast
         brace (see Neufeld
         traction)
   splints, 83-84
   with traction splint and Pear-
         son attachment, for
         proximal tibial skeletal
         traction, 81-88
Balanced suspension with double
         slings, 89-93
   for fractures of the distal
         two-thirds of the
         femoral shaft, 89
   for fractures of lower third
         of femur, 92
   for proximal tibial skeletal
         traction, 90
Bite block, Cotrel traction, 30
Bohler's angle, effects of cal-
         caneal traction, 98

Bohler-Steinmann pin bows, for
         distal tibial skeletal
         traction, 95
Bradford frame, 5-7
   for pelvic or acetabular frac-
         tures, 63
   with pelvic sling suspension
         for pelvic fractures, 61
Buck's extension
   dislocation of the hip, 67
   for femoral fractures, 67-68
   for low back pain, 67
   for nondisplaced acetabular
         fractures, 67
   skin traction, 67
Buck's traction
   for acetabular fracture, 62
   uphill or high angle, for
         femoral shaft fracture
         in a small child, 72
   with sling (see Split Russell's
         traction)
Bryant's traction, low angle
   for shaft fracture in infant
         or small child, 72
   Volkmann's contracture, risk
         of, 72

C

Calcaneal traction, 98, 99
   for calcaneal fracture, indi-
         cations and disadvan-
         tages, 98
   loss of tuber joint (Bohler's)
         angle, 98
   pin insertion, preferred site,
         98, 100

Cervical traction, 15-29
  excessive manipulation of head,
      spinal injury from, 21
  halo ring traction, 23-29
  head halter traction, 15-18,
      22-23
  home management, 24
  laceration of scalp, 21
  outpatient, for chronic neck
      pain, 22
  skeletal, 18-29
  tongs, types and application
      techniques, 18-22
Cervicogenic arm, head halter
      traction, 15
Chinese finger traps, 56
Circulatory embarrassment, to
      fingers, in skin
      traction, 45
Clavicle fracture, simple fore-
      arm skin traction,
      43-45
Colles' fracture, finger trap
      traction for, 56
Compartment syndromes
  overhead olecranon pin traction,
      52
  tibial, 98
Cotrel traction, 30-31
  bite block, 30
  dynamic, 30
  Harrington rod instrumentation,
      30
  low back pain, 30
  scoliosis, 30
  spinal deformities, 30-31
Crutchfield tongs, for cervical
      traction, 18, 21-22

D

DiCosola rope holders, 83
Dunlop's skin traction, for lar-
      ger child in a fracture
      bed, 49
Dunlop's traction
  for child in crib, 49
  for supracondylar and trans-
      condylar fractures in
      children, 48-50

Dynamic dorsiflexor, 88
Dynamic traction, Cotrel, 30

E

Equipment (see Orthopaedic equip-
      ment and the specific
      device)
Extremities (see Lower extremity
      traction; Upper extre-
      mity traction)

F

Femoral fractures, 67-79
  balanced suspension with double
      slings, 89
  Buck's extension, 67-68
  low angle Bryant's traction, 72
  lower third, balanced suspension
      with double slings, 92
  middle and distal thirds, split
      Russell's traction, in
      children, 69
  90-90° traction through distal
      femur, 72-76
  proximal third, 73
  proximal tibial traction in ex-
      tension, 79
  subtrochanteric, 73
  uphill or high angle Buck's
      traction, 72
Femoral fractures, distal two-
      thirds
  balanced suspension with double
      slings, 89
  balanced suspension with trac-
      tion splint and Pearson
      attachment, 81
  Neufeld traction combined with
      proximal tibial trac-
      tion, 93-94
  proximal tibial skeletal trac-
      tion, 81
Femoral skeletal traction, upper
      eyelet screw, 63
  for acetabular fractures, 62-65
Femoral traction, distal, in ex-
      tension, 77-79
  equipment, 81

for fractures of pelvis or aceta-
     bulum, 77-79
Femoral traction, halo (see Halo
     femoral traction)
Femoral trochanteric traction,
     proximal, for acetabular
     fracture, 65
Finger trap traction, 56-57
  Chinese finger traps, 56
  for Colles' fracture, 56
Flexion contracture, 90-90 degrees
     traction through distal
     femur, 73

                G

Gardner tongs, for cervical
     traction, 18-21

                H

Halo brace, 27
Halo femoral traction, 30-33
  for spinal deformities, 30-33
  for stabilizing a thoracic
       spinal fracture, 32
  Harrington rod instrumentation,
       32
  lateral rectus muscle palsy, 32
  neurological examinations, 32
  Stryker frame, 32
Halo pelvic traction, for spinal
     deformities, 32-36
Halo ring traction
  cervical, 23-29
  low profile halo, 29
  lumbar spine deformity, 34
  pin cleaning, 27
  pin penetration, 29
  pin sites, 29
  pins, 23, 25
  plastic jacket, 25, 27, 28
  pressure sores, 29
  risks, 29
  Risser frame, 27
  sizes of ring, 23
  spinal deformities, 23-29, 34
  thoracic spine deformity, 34
  with pelvic girdle, 34
Halo suspension traction, 36-37

for spinal deformities, 36-37
in wheelchair, 37
on incline bed, 37
Stagnara's, 36
Harrington rod instrumentation
  Cotrel traction, 30
  halo femoral traction, 32
Head halter traction, 15-18,
     22-23
  excessive weight, injuries
       from, 17
  frame, in hospital bed, 17
  on a Stryker frame, 16
  outpatient, 22-23
Hip and knee exerciser, 71
Hip, dislocation, Buck's ex-
     tension, 67
Hoffman type fixation
  for proximal tibial traction in
       extension, 81
Humeral fractures
  distal, overhead olecranon pin
       traction, 50
  lateral olecranon pin traction,
       53
Humeral shaft fractures, proximal,
     double skin traction,
     46-48

                I

Ischemic contracture, in trans-
     condylar or supra-
     condylar fracture, 50

                K

Knee and hip exerciser, 71
Knots, 11-13
  clove hitch, 11
  overhand loop, 11-12
  slip knot, 11, 13

                L

Lower extremity traction, 67-104
  balanced suspensions, 81-98
  calcaneal, 98
  femoral, 67-79
  knee and hip exerciser, 71

low angle Bryant's traction,
        72
split Russell's traction, 69-71
tibial, 79-88
transmetatarsal suspension, 98
Lumbar spine deformity, halo
        ring traction, 34
Lumbar traction, 38-40
  home pelvic traction, 38-40
  inpatient pelvic belt, 38-40

                    M

Metacarpal pin traction, 54-56
  pin placement, 55
  sling counterweight, balanced,
        55

                    N

Neck injury, head halter traction
        for, 15
Neck pain
  head halter traction, 15-18
  outpatient head halter traction,
        22-23
Neufeld cast brace
  complications from, 94
  for proximal tibial skeletal
        traction, 95
  polycentric hinges, 94
Neufeld traction, combined with
        proximal tibial trac-
        tion, for fractures of
        the distal two-thirds
        of the femoral shaft,
        93-94
Ninety-90 degree traction through
        distal femur, 72-76
  flexion contracture, 73
  for fractures of proximal third
        of femoral shaft, 73
  for subtrochanteric fractures,
        73
  support sling, 75-76
  traction pin insertion, pre-
        ferred site, 75

                    O

Olecranon pin traction (lateral),

        53-54
  for humeral fractures, 53
  shallow pin placement, 53
Olecranon pin traction (overhead)
        50-53
  compartment syndromes, 52
  for fractures of distal humerus,
        50
  for supracondylar fractures, 50
Orthopaedic equipment, 5-10
  beds and frames, 5-10
  pole fittings, 8
  pulleys, 9
  weights (sandbags, cast iron,
        water bags), 9-10

                    P

Pearson attachment
  for balanced suspension with
        traction splint, 81-88
  for proximal tibial traction
        in extension, 81
Pelvic belt traction
  inpatient, for conservative
        treatment of low back
        pain, 38
Pelvic or acetabular fracture
  Bradford frame, 63
  Buck's traction, 62
  distal femoral traction in
        extension, 77-79
  fracture bed for, 63
  pelvic sling suspension for
        pelvic fractures, 61-62
  proximal femoral trochanteric
        traction, 65
  Russell's traction, 62
  upper femoral skeletal traction
        for acetabular fractures
        62-65
Pelvic sling suspension
  for pelvic fractures, 61-62
  with Bradford frame, 61
Pelvic traction
  halo, for spinal deformities,
        32-36
  home management, 38, 40
Peroneal nerve palsy, caused by
        Buck's traction, 69

Plastic jacket, halo ring traction, 25, 27, 28
Pressure sores, halo ring traction, 29

R

Rectus muscle palsy, caused by halo femoral traction, 32
Risser frame, for halo ring traction, 27
Rotator cuff impingement, in simple forearm skin traction, 45
Russell's traction
  for acetabular fractures, 62
  split (see Split Russell's traction)

S

Scoliosis, Cotrel traction, 30
Shoulder paid, head halter traction, 15
Skeletal traction, to distal femur, 77
Skin traction, 43-48
  Buck's extension, 67
  Dunlop's, for child in a fracture bed, 49
  yokes available for, 46
Skin traction, double (forearm and upper arm), 46-48
  for proximal humeral shaft fractures, 46-48
Skin traction, simple forearm, 43-45
  circulatory embarrassment to fingers, 45
  for clavicle fracture, 43-45
  rotator cuff impingement, 45
  skin loss, 45
Skull traction, for spinal deformith, 23
Spinal traction, 15-41
  cervical, 15-29
  lumbar, 38-40
  spinal deformities, 29-37
Spine, unstable, cervical skeletal traction, 18-29
Splints

hinged half-ring, 83
full ring, 83
Thomas, 83
Split Russell's traction, 69-71
  for fractures of the middle and distal thirds of the femur in children, 69
Stagnara halo suspension traction, 36
Stryker frame
  with halo femoral traction, 32
  with head halter traction, 16
Supracondylar fractures
  Dunlop's technique, 48-50
  ischemic (or Volkmann's) contracture, 50
  overhead olecranon pin traction, 50

T

Thomas splint, 83
Thoracic spine deformity, halo ring traction, 34
Thoracic spine fracture, stabilization, with halo femoral traction, 32
Tibial compartment pressure syndrome, complicating distal tibial skeletal traction, 98
Tibial plateau fractures, distal tibial skeletal traction, 95
Tibial shaft fractures, temporary immobilization with distal tibial skeletal traction, 97
Tibial skeletal traction, distal, 94-98
  Bohler-Steinmann pin bows, 95
  for temporary immobilization of tibial shaft fracture, 97
  for tibial plateau fractures, 95
  tibial compartment pressure syndrome, 98

traction pin insertion through
        distal tibia and
        fibula, 97
Tibial skeletal traction, proximal
  balanced suspension in double
        splints, 90
  balanced suspension with
        traction splint and
        Pearson attachment, 81-88
  for fractures of the distal
        two-thirds of the
        femur, 81
  with cast brace (Neufeld), 95
Tibial traction, proximal, in
        extension, 79-82
  cast brace for, 81
  equipment, 81
  for fractures of distal two-
        thirds of femoral
        shaft, 79
  Hoffman type external fixation,
        81
  Pearson attachment, 81
  wire insertion, preferred site,
        80
Transcondylar fractures
  Dunlop's technique, 48-50
  ischemic (or Volkmann's)
        contracture, 50
Transmetatarsal suspension, 98-99,
        101
  and transtibial suspension, for
        burn treatment and pre-
        vention of plantar
        flexion contracture, 101
  joint of Lisfranc in, 99
  pin traction infection, 99
Tuber joint (Bohler's) angle,
        loss of, with calcaneal
        traction, 98

                  U

Upper extremity traction, 43-59
  Dunlop's technique, 48-50
  finger trap traction, 56-57
  metacarpal pin traction, 54-56
  olecranon pin traction, 50-54
  skin traction, 43-48

                  V

Vascular obstruction, caused by
        Buck's extension, 69
Veneke tongs, for cervical
        traction, 18
Volkmann's contracture
  in transcondylar or supra-
        condylar fracture, 50
  risk of, with low angle
        Bryant's traction, 72

                  W

Wheelchair, halo traction, 37